The Crisis of Chronic Disease among Aboriginal Peoples: A Challenge for Public Health, Population Health and Social Policy

J. Reading Ph.D. | Director, Centre for Aboriginal Health Research

Special thanks to Andrew Kmetic and all of the people who contributed to the creation and editing of this book: Ekaterina Bruic, Daniell De Jong, Elizabeth Estey, Ashley Heaslip, Miranda Kelly, Dinara Kurbanova, Rachel Link, Namaste Marsden, Geoff McKee, Colleen O'Leary, Josh Haneul Seo and Megan Stepushyn

Centre for Aboriginal Health Research | University of Victoria, British Columbia, Canada

---

University of Victoria Centre for Aboriginal Health Research acknowledges its funders:

CIHR IRSC
Canadian Institutes of Health Research | Instituts de recherche en santé du Canada

University of Victoria

Network Environments for Aboriginal Research BC

Michael Smith Foundation for Health Research

ISBN 978-1-55058-407-3

Contents

Part I: A Message from the Director

Now is the time to tackle a growing challenge, that of improving the health and well being of Aboriginal peoples in Canada.

It is no secret that Aboriginal peoples in Canada, no matter where they live, face unique health challenges. They experience higher rates of diabetes, heart disease, tuberculosis, HIV/AIDS and many other diseases. Infant mortality rates are higher and life expectancy is lower than in the general population. The Aboriginal suicide rate is two-to-three times higher than the non-Aboriginal rate for Canada and, within the youth age group, this rate is estimated to be five-to-six times higher.

Aboriginal young people are being encouraged to take up health research as a career, as a vocation and as a way to improve the lives of their people.

And, because many of the health challenges that Aboriginal peoples face are strikingly similar the world over, research needs to work closely with Indigenous communities and health research organizations in Australia, New Zealand, the United States, circumpolar northern nations and low and middle income countries to develop collaborative approaches to investigate and find solutions to these complex health challenges (Centre for Aboriginal Health Research, 2009).

A great deal has been done to investigate factors that describe the health of Aboriginal peoples living in Canada through research. Community based interventions are now needed to focus policies and strategies, to ensure that we are making meaningful, long-term improvements across a wide range of health issues facing Aboriginal peoples.

Aboriginal community health professionals, funding agencies, governments and researchers need to identify new, innovative and transformative ideas from the broader Indigenous community, where the aim is to improve health if critical problems are better understood.

This book is an examination of Aboriginal Health throughout the life course. Each section is divided into areas where specific indicators are compared and explained in terms of their potential to improve health through intervention. The idea is to identify pressing health priorities and to use evidence to inform innovative programs targeted to addressing health concerns. Interventions need rigorous evaluation to assess program success so managers can improve the intervention and to share the results with other communities who may need to create similar programs in other communities. This book is intended to help inform students, community researchers, government and non-governmental organizations, and the public who want to understand the health of Aboriginal peoples.

To facilitate collaborative research ventures, the Canadian Institutes of Health Research have published Guidelines for Health Research Involving Aboriginal Peoples (CIHR, 2007). The idea is to engage community collectives in a transition from the previous role of research subjects to that of actively engaged research participants and leaders.

The ground breaking public policy focuses on Aboriginal health research ethics guidelines, in particular research partnership methodology; collective and individual consent; protection of cultural knowledge; benefit sharing; and collection, use, storage and secondary use of data and biological samples. Through the development of research agreements, communities can engage in research and over time, a foundation of trust is expected to develop between Aboriginal communities and researchers. Research ethics boards need to improve their competence in reviewing research proposals that involve Aboriginal communities while Aboriginal communities take a greater role in initiating, understanding and directing their autonomous research activities. The ultimate goals are to improve the health and well being of Aboriginal peoples through community based research that builds on the traditional health practices of Aboriginal communities and develops innovative programs and services, which better meet the needs of Aboriginal people.

While the approaches being taken today are valuable and will result in improved health for Aboriginal peoples living in Canada, it is time for a bolder approach that takes into consideration the entire life course. For example, an international longitudinal cohort study of Aboriginal child health could elucidate factors related to improved health outcomes for vulnerable communities. The idea is to develop a model to optimize the developmental trajectory of vulnerable children at each stage throughout the entire life course, beginning with improving the health of young women through a pre-conception intervention. This would be followed seamlessly by age and gender specific interventions along the life course continuum through infancy, early childhood or pre-school years, childhood and youth, adult and Elders. Collectively, we need to use the research enterprise to find solutions to pressing gaps in health and well being for Aboriginal peoples living in Canada and abroad.

A second example in this book is to look at chronic diseases among Aboriginal peoples; including cancer, heart health, diabetes, mental health and addictions with relevance to prevention, intervention, health services, rehabilitation and emergency primary care.

A key to using research to develop new health programs is specifically embedding a process for knowledge translation into all Aboriginal health research. This recognizes that policy makers are critical to success of improving health through new evidence based programs and need to be involved in a knowledge translation process to ensure that new ideas can be the basis for innovative programs and policies which aim for improving Aboriginal health.

Aboriginal peoples' health needs to shape Canada's research agenda, focusing attention on the critical areas that could, once fully understood, contribute to improve Aboriginal peoples' health. Such an approach might focus on finding innovation in areas that include but are not limited to:

- Preventing diseases, such as diabetes, heart disease, HIV/AIDS, tuberculosis and many other conditions described in the book;
- Improving quality of life such as provision of adequate community infrastructure such as housing and clean water;
- Addressing factors associated with equitable provision of health services, including public health or health care delivery approaches across the entire spectrum of the health care system;
- Examining broad social policy issues, such as eradication of poverty, access to educational opportunities or improvement to early childhood development; and
- Addressing knowledge gaps in the complex and sensitive areas of mental health, addictions, suicide prevention and issues of violence, criminal justice and healthy sexuality.

Aboriginal communities are resilient. In the face of challenging obstacles a growing number of communities have created healthy environments and sustainable economic opportunities for their people. The promising practices of communities need to be shared among and between communities to promote health for future generations.

The challenge is for researchers to work with the Aboriginal communities defining the opportunities that can transform health and that demands the involvement of the most creative and informed minds, both Aboriginal and non-Aboriginal, in Canada.

The health of Aboriginal peoples living in Canada is not going to improve overnight. But it must improve if Aboriginal communities are to share in and contribute to Canada's prosperity and development.

Part II: Chronic Disease Risk Factors in Aboriginal peoples in Canada – A Life Course Approach

1. Introduction: Taking a Life course Approach

In order to stem the rise of chronic diseases in developed countries throughout the twentieth century, and particularly in the post-war period, epidemiologists, health care professionals, and policy makers targeted adult risk factors. Thus, targeting adult behaviour and lifestyle factors, such as obesity, smoking, and high cholesterol became the prevailing model for the prevention and intervention of chronic disease (Kuh & Ben-Shlomo, 2004). In the developed world, this approach and its programs have been very successful in alleviating problems associated with chronic diseases: results from the 40-year Framingham heart study indicate that in the United States, more than one-half of the decline in coronary heart disease mortality observed in women and one-third to one-half of the decline observed in men can be attributed to changes in adult risk factors (Sytkowski, D'Agostino, Belanger, & Kannel, 1996). Unfortunately, the overall improvement in adult risk factors and chronic disease is limited to certain populations: while rates of some chronic disease have declined in Western populations, chronic diseases are a growing cause of mortality and morbidity among vulnerable populations, like Aboriginal peoples (Smeja & Brassard, 2000).

Another problem with the adult risk factor approach is that, while adults are being targeted to change their lifestyle habits, the next generation will grow up in the same conditions that have fostered the development and onset of chronic disease in their parents. When these conditions are grounded in poor socioeconomic status, the disease risk is increased and the applications of an adult lifestyle approach to chronic disease is ineffective. Social disparities and inequities in health documented in Aboriginal communities across the country suggest that an adult risk factors approach alone is not enough. Results from recent Aboriginal studies reinforce a "determinants of health framework," which indicates that broader social-welfare provisions must be considered in the fight to reduce disparities in health (Newbold, 1998).

In the last 20 years, life course epidemiology has emerged as an alternative approach to the prevailing adult risk model described above (Kuh, Ben-

Shlomo, Lynch, Hallqvist, & Power, 2003). Life course epidemiology has been defined as the study of long-term effects of physical or social exposures during gestation, childhood, adolescence, young adulthood, and adult life on one's developmental health and later disease risk (Kuh, et al., 2003). Life course epidemiology offers a way to conceptualize how underlying biological and socio-environmental determinants of health, experienced at different life course stages, can differentially influence the development of chronic diseases (Moore & Davies, 2005). The benefit of this perspective is that it expands the conventional adult lifestyle models of disease risk by recognizing that psychosocial, as well as physiological factors occurring throughout an individual's life can affect a diverse range of outcomes, from general well-being to physical functioning and the development of chronic disease (Ben-Shlomo & Kuh, 2002; CDC, 1996; Darnton-Hill, Nishida, & James, 2004). A major strength of this approach is that it also shows how risks occurring throughout life can be identified, corrected, and/or modified over the long time frame it takes for chronic diseases to develop (Lynch & Smith, 2005). In a parallel manner, Danton-Hill describes a life course perspective as allowing "one to see health differences among populations, social classes, etc. as resulting from an accumulation of material disadvantages [and] that reflect widely differing economic and social life circumstances". Only after thinking of disease as an aspect of an individual's life course can "the prevention and control of chronic diseases…be intimately integrated into normal daily life", and sustained to benefit the health of communities. Thus, strategies that address risk factors must continually account for "the underlying economic, gender, political, behavioural and environmental factors that foster these disease risks" (Darnton-Hill, et al., 2004) within all age groups and across generations.

What the life course approach also adds to the adult risk factor model is an understanding of and attention to timing and the duration of exposures to risks (Ben-Shlomo & Kuh, 2002). There are a number of models that have been used to account for the importance of timing in disease development and used as a basis for underlying theoretical frameworks for life course studies. The ***critical period model*** assumes that exposure at a certain period, usually early in life, has a permanent effect that remains relatively stable throughout an individual's life. This model can be extended by considering the interaction of these early exposures with exposures later in life. Another possible model is the ***accumulation of risks model*** that posits the development of disease as a result of cumulative exposure and damage over the life course to some threshold. Finally, there is a ***pathway model*** that suggests that exposure increases the likelihood of further exposure, which can eventually result in the development of a disease. While the emphasis on exposure time, magnitude, and impact is different for each of these models, they all speak to the importance of engaging with the interconnection between time and disease risk in order to chart a better understanding of the etiology of chronic diseases. In addition to the benefit of life course for the organization and investigation methods of research, a life course approach provides an effective tool for policy makers. This is because, as the World Health Organization (WHO) notes, a life course approach can help identify the most effective and potentially successful policies and prevention methods for chronic diseases (WHO, 2005a). As this book attempts to demonstrate, the life course approach is also a good organizational tool and method to review and assess the current state of the literature on important health topics.

1.1 The Life Course Perspective and Aboriginal Health

The burden of chronic diseases among Aboriginal peoples, described and discussed in Part III of this book, is a serious public health concern. As the morbidity and mortality rates related to chronic diseases continue to show signs of growth in this population (Smeja & Brassard, 2000; Thomas, et al., 2006), a new approach to studying disease trends and facilitating positive interventions is urgently needed. As described above, the life course perspective provides one appropriate theoretical model to do this. Further still, the life course approach is complementary to Aboriginal perspectives on health.

Specifically, benefits of a life course perspective in the context of Aboriginal communities are twofold; First, the method provides researchers with the tools to integrate scientific, cultural, and sociological knowledge in a meaningful way; this fusion is necessary to satisfy both the scientific and cultural requirements of Aboriginal health research. Secondly, life course research understands health in a holistic way (Lynch & Smith, 2005), which complements Aboriginal conceptions of health and well-being that encompass the physical, mental, emotional, and spiritual domains (Bartlett, 1998; Isaak & Marchessault, 2008). This is exemplified by a quote from the 2002/03 First Nations Regional Longitudinal Health Survey (RHS): "The medicine wheel life cycle connects the experiences and wellness of infants to the experiences and wellness of children, youth, young adults, parents, grandparents, and elders, again from an individual, family, community, and First Nations perspective" (First Nations Centre, 2005).

The crisis in Aboriginal peoples' health today is complicated by issues that are deeply rooted in social disparities (Adelson, 2005), which is why there is concern that *no amount of risk assessment or health recommendations will reduce the burden of disease without a parallel understanding of the importance of social change.* Life course epidemiology offers a conceptual framework to integrate social and biological risk factors (Kuh, et al., 2003): it allows the researcher and the community to map out the dominant risk patterns in their region and target their eradication before an accumulation of those risks becomes a problem. Since research that is "by and for" Aboriginal peoples and reflects Aboriginal perspectives is the most likely to improve the health of Aboriginal peoples (J. O'Neil, Reading, Bartlett, Young, & Kaufert, 1999), life course approach's recognition of social and cultural values is also promising. As different Aboriginal populations gradually acquire the resources necessary for their empowerment, the applications of life course epidemiology could have the potential to be used in novel prevention-intervention-based policy recommendations.

1.2 Applying the life course approach

By studying an individual's development and exposures to risks throughout the life course, in terms of biological conditions and socioeconomic factors, chronic disease patterns can be better understood. In order to apply this mentality, this book's discussion of chronic disease risk factors will be organized through a life course perspective. Thus, the risk factors noted in the literature will be discussed in the particular life stage that they have a profound impact or at which they place an individual at the greatest risk for developing chronic diseases. This section will begin, however, with a discussion of the community-level or broad reaching risk factors that influence health and well-being across the life course. These cross-cutting risk factors are discussed first to help set the stage and highlight the underlining factors influencing the health and well-being of the Aboriginal population. Following this, this section will begin to look at the specific life stages. Naturally, this will begin with a discussion of prenatal risk factors. It will follow with in-depth discussions of natal, early childhood,

childhood and adolescent, and adulthood risk factors. This seems like a natural and logical ordering that follows the life trajectory and temporal course of risk exposure(s) and disease development. While this separation of the different life stages is important, it is also important to remember that many risk factors are present at multiple life stages. To avoid duplication, the importance of the timing of the exposure and the impact of risk factors on long-term health and development will be given attention.

A broad determinants of health perspective will also ground the discussion of the context in which risk factors flourish or decline. That is, biological, social, economic, environmental, and political factors that affect one's health, and the health of communities, populations, and generations will all be included. This will enable a broad discussion of the complex and strikingly similar risk factor environments for Indigenous populations globally.

2. Community Risk Factors

Community risk factors are defined and discussed here as those that have impact health at multiple life stages, beyond an individual's life span, across a generation, and between generations. These multi-level factors are an important addition to the traditional risk factor model: thinking of risk factors as they act across and within generations is important because it encourages the consideration of collective health issues and the interconnections that exist between health and society. This will prepare the reader for discussions of the Aboriginal health research environment, and how the efforts of the Canadian government to oppress the cultures, traditions, and community structures of Aboriginal peoples has caused collective trauma and grief that is thought to have cumulated as health problems in many Aboriginal communities (First Nations Centre, 2005; Kirmayer, Brass, & Tait, 2000). In addition to the social, political, cultural, and academic history of Aboriginal health, this chapter will examine the community risk factors associated with socioeconomic status and geography. This focus is important because it will enable a rich discussion of the social determinants of health that act on communities and collectives and impact the health and well-being of such communities. This is particularly important to do with regards to the prevalence of chronic diseases, where social, economic, and environmental issues have been shown to have a profound effect on disease risk and mortality (NSW Health, 2006).

2.1 Socioeconomic Risk Factors

The ill health of Aboriginal peoples has been linked to "the corrosive effects of poverty and economic marginalization" (Kirmayer, et al., 2000), but these social determinants of health have themselves been described as both direct and indirect consequences of historic policies of colonization (First Nations Centre, 2005; King, 2006). As such, the risks associated with colonization are interrelated and connected to the risks posed by socio-economic disadvantage (Beauchamp, et al., 2004; Carson, Dunbar, Chenhall, & Bailie, 2007; Health Canada, 2003; Reading, Kmetic, & Gideon, 2007). Unfortunately, Indigenous peoples worldwide are disproportionately burdened with disease risk from such social determinants as poverty, low household incomes, and lack of adequate (or no) housing (Adelson, 2005; Beauchamp, et al., 2004; Canada, 2006; First Nations Centre, 2005; Health Canada, 2003). Since "social inequality, whether measured at the population or individual level, is the single leading condition for poor health" (Geyorfi-Dyke, 2008), such social disadvantages highlight the risks placed on the health and well-being of Aboriginal peoples. The potential impact of socioeconomic factors is even more obvious when one considers the burden placed on the biological development of individuals as these disadvantages accumulate across the life-course and across generations (Adelson, 2005; Beauchamp, et al., 2004; Carson, et al., 2007; M. G. Marmot & Wilkinson, 1999; Warry, 1998). It is from this perspective that the specific influence of poverty and socioeconomic status, as well as housing, on chronic disease development is discussed below.

2.1.1 Low Socioeconomic Status and Poverty

While child poverty will be briefly discussed in the "early childhood risk factors" (part II section 5, pg 45-51); the impacts of poverty and poor socioeconomic status (SES) on chronic diseases are included here to emphasize the intergenerational and cyclical nature of poverty: child poverty is family poverty, is community poverty, is generational poverty. That is, poverty rarely affects just one individual, at one time, but is an issue that transcends age and time.

Defining and Describing Poverty for Aboriginal peoples in Canada

While poverty can (and has) been described and defined in a number of different ways, it is often classified according to its extremity. As such, it is often labelled as: extreme, moderate, and relative poverty. *Extreme poverty* is when households (or individuals) cannot meet their basic needs for survival. *Moderate poverty* is when basic needs are barely met. And, finally, *relative poverty* is when the household income is less than the national average income (WHO, 2008c). Thus, relative poverty is often equated with the terms "low income" and "poor/low socioeconomic status." In Canada, relative poverty, or low income, is measured using Low-Income Cut-Offs (LICOs) developed by Statistics Canada (Ross, Shillington, & Lochhead, 1994; Statistics Canada, 1999a). Despite the presence of varied experiences, measures, and approaches, it is clear that all types of poverty adversely affect one's health. As such, this section will discuss the general connection between poverty and chronic diseases. First, however, the prevalence of poverty among Aboriginal populations will be reviewed.

To measure and compare the quality of life between different countries or populations, the United Nations developed the Human Development Index (HDI). This index has been applied in Canada in an effort to compare the quality of life and well-being of Aboriginal and non-Aboriginal people (INAC, 2004). Canada has been consistently ranked according to the HDI as one of the top five countries in the world. When the HDI rank is controlled for Aboriginal ancestry, however, registered Indian peoples living on reserve in Canada ranked a shockingly low 78th place. This score is on par with countries such as Peru (79th) and Brazil (80th) (Blackstock, 2005). This is demonstrated by the gap between the lines in Figure 1. The figure also demonstrates that: (1) the HDI score for both Registered Indians and other Canadians has increased from 1981 to 2001; (2) the gap in HDI scores has reduced (from 0.146 in 1991 to 0.115 in 2001), and (3) a large discrepancy between the health of Registered Indians and other Canadians clearly and profoundly remains. It should also be noted that although similar trends exist, the overall gap is even greater between Inuit and other Canadians (from 0.159 in 1991 to 0.142 in 2001) (INAC). This highlights the often-sighted analogy that Aboriginal Peoples in Canada are living in Third World conditions within a First World country (O'Neill, 2007).

Figure 1. The Human Development Index for Registered Indians and Other Canadians, 1981-2001

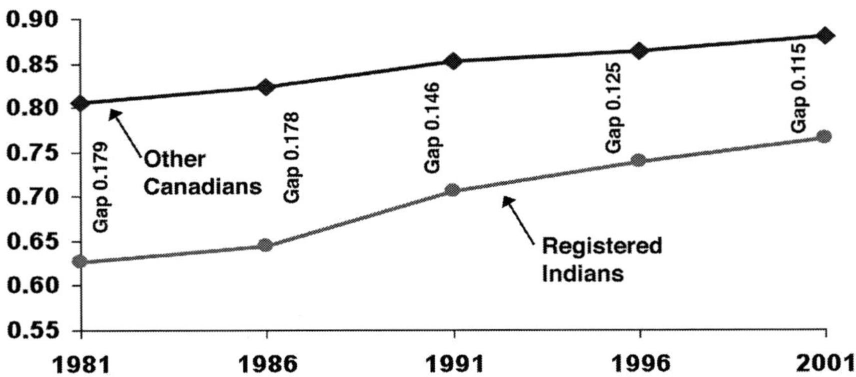

Source: (INAC, 2004).

In addition to the HDI, income statistics and poverty rates exemplify the poor SES of many Aboriginal peoples. For example, "47.2% of the Ontario Aboriginal population receives less than $10,000 per year" (Ontario Federation of Indian Friendship Centres, 2004). Canada-wide statistics also show that Aboriginal people are economically disadvantaged: 73.4% of Aboriginal people earn < $20,000 per year, and the average income is $ 15,699 versus $25,414 in the rest of Canada (Sin, Wells, Svenson, & Man, 2002). Information collected in urban settings demonstrates that this subset of the Aboriginal population is significantly disadvantaged compared to their non-Aboriginal counterparts. For example, a study done in 2000 reported that Aboriginal peoples living in urban settings are twice as likely to live in poverty than non-Aboriginal people. Further, while accounting for only 1.5% of the urban population, Aboriginal peoples account for 3.4% of the poor population (Lee, 2000).

Poverty and Health

As has been demonstrated elsewhere and will be discussed in the life stage discussions, traditional adult risk factors, such as smoking, high blood pressure, obesity, and poor diet, are common and concerning risk factors for the development of chronic diseases. However, such risk factors only explain a fraction of the incidence and prevalence of chronic disease and the mortality from such diseases in Aboriginal populations. For instance, research has continually shown that SES can have a profound impact on the prevalence and mortality of disease (M. G. Marmot, Kogevinas, & Elston, 1987; Smith, Hart, Blane, Gillis, & Hawthorne, 1997; Smye & Browne, 2002; S. L. Syme, 2004; van Rossum, Shipley, van de Mheen, Grobbee, & Marmot, 2000): there exists "abundant data showing a link between poverty and ill health" (Marmot & Wilkinson, 1999). For instance, it has been noted that "the higher the socio-economic level of the household the lower the mortality rate" (Marmot, 2005). Research has found that traditional adult risk factors can only account for approximately 25-35% of the mortality associated with this "social gradient" (Marmot, 2005; S. L. Syme, 1989). While all aspects of this association have yet to be determined, research documenting the relationship between poverty and chronic disease prevalence and mortality will be discussed below.

Poverty increases an individual's, a family's, and a community's risk of developing chronic diseases, developing complications, and dying (WHO, 2008c). This is because material deprivation, unhealthy living conditions (e.g. poor housing, inadequate food supply), and poor access to heath care services predispose people with low SES to the development of chronic diseases and the uptake of risk behaviours throughout the life course (NSW Health, 2006). For instance, WHO notes that "the poor and people with less education are more likely to use tobacco products and to consume energy-dense and high-fat food, be physically inactive, and be overweight or obese" (WHO, 2008c). Psychosocial stress is also considered to be a major contributor to the ill health of those living in poverty. Notable researchers, such as Marmot and Syme, discuss such stress as the *loss of one's control over their destiny* and, therefore, their ability to deal with the forces that affect their day-to-day lives is a key component of the link between SES and health (M. G. Marmot, 2005; M. G. Marmot & Swan, 1998; S. L. Syme, 1989, 2004; S. L. Syme & Swan, 1998). This theory has been supported by research that has found that "control of destiny" is lower in the lower status groups (Marmot, 2005). Neuroendocrinological studies have also shown that lack of control over life circumstances creates stress load on the body, which is thought to contribute to the development of a variety of diseases and conditions, especially insulin dependent diabetes, cardiovascular diseases (McEwan & Swan, 1998; McEwen, 2006), alcoholism, and suicide (S. L. Syme & Swan, 1998). In addition to the imposition of stress and loss of control over one's future, stress related to finances, lack of access to healthy food or any food at all, lack of access to basic health care, poor living conditions, and inability to provide basic needs; all demonstrate the correlation between poor SES and health (Behrman, 1995). While there is reason to be encouraged by the fact that the SES of many Aboriginal peoples has increased in recent years, a gap between Aboriginal and non-Aboriginal people remains (see Figure 1). The same is often true for Indigenous populations around the world: Indigenous populations in developed countries are "a socially excluded minority within their countries" (Marmot, 2005) and "over-represented in lower SES strata" (Valery, Coory, Stirling, & Green, 2006). The direct impact of the overrepresentation of Aboriginal peoples in the lower SES categories affects mental health, cancer, and respiratory disease are presented as examples of specific chronic disease impacts.

Socioeconomic disparities and, particularly, their relationship to a loss of control of destiny are a major risk factor for mental health problems (Canada, 2006a; Warry, 1998). As Warry (1998) explains, problems of alcohol abuse and family violence among Aboriginal peoples are deeply rooted in a perceived lack of control over life. Syme (2004) suggested that a lack of "control of destiny" contributes to community-level health problems and interferes with the desire among Aboriginal peoples to assume responsibility for their health and well-being (Warry, 1998). For instance, some severely mentally ill individuals have identified poverty as having a debilitating impact on their self-esteem, social networking, leisure activities, and abilities to meet their basic needs, visit their family members, and form intimate relationships (Wilton, 2004). The debilitation from poverty is often thought to be more difficult to deal with than the diagnosis or ongoing treatment of the disease itself. And, issues related to poverty tend to exacerbate the intensity, persistence, and effects of the disease (Lee, 2000).

The relationship between SES and cancer risk is very complex. This is because current research reports that having a higher SES can predispose people to some types of cancer (e.g. lung, breast, colorectal), while having a lower SES can place people at risk for other types of cancer (e.g. stomach, liver, and cervical) (Brown, Goldie, Draisma, Harford, & Lipscomb, 2006). Comparisons between developed and developing countries, which has led to these conclusions, can, in part, be translatable to the study of the origins of Aboriginal cancer risk in Canada, as Aboriginal people have been likened to developing societies that live within a developed country (Epstein, 1982). And, as the prevalence of cancer in Aboriginal populations shows, the so called "third world cancers" are generally more common in Aboriginal peoples than are the "Western cancers." This suggests that targeting the SES, as a risk factor may help to alleviate certain types of cancer risk among Aboriginal peoples. Clearly, more attention needs to be given to the interaction between poverty and cancer risk throughout the life course. Attention to the role that income has on the burden of cancer in Aboriginal peoples is also important as low SES has been shown to lead to decreased cancer survival rates (L. D. Marrett & Chaudhry, 2003).

Socioeconomic status has also been shown to impact the prevalence of diabetes. A 2003 study found substantial clustering of diabetes in areas of Winnipeg with low SES, poor environmental quality, poor lifestyles and a high concentration of Aboriginal people (Green, Hoppa, Young, & Blanchard, 2003). The study found that education and income were stronger predictors of diabetes than Aboriginal status, suggesting that socioeconomic status, rather than genetic factors were responsible for the high prevalence of diabetes (Green, Hoppa, et al., 2003). Despite studies that demonstrate potential correlations between poverty and health, it is important to remember that *poverty alone does not determine the health of an individual or population.* Thus, the complete nature of the relationship between poverty and illness, and in particular chronic diseases, in Aboriginal populations has yet to be determined and should be the focus of further research. This should include an examination of poverty as a risk factor for chronic disease development, as well as chronic diseases as a risk factor for poverty. This is because:

> *Chronic diseases inflict an enormous direct and indirect economic burden on the poor, and push many people and their families into poverty. Further, the death or illness of parents or caring adults can lead to the impoverishment of their children and/or their community. Existing knowledge underestimates the implications of chronic diseases for poverty and the potential that chronic disease prevention and health promotion have for alleviating poverty (WHO, 2008c).*

As this quote highlights, the prevention of chronic diseases and interventions targeting underlying social determinants of health have the bi-directional potential to greatly improve poverty rates and contribute to the general well-being of Aboriginal peoples.

2.1.2 Shelter and Housing

In addition to and interrelated with issues of income are issues related to shelter. Like income, housing disadvantages have been acknowledged as having potentially negative health impacts (Carson, Dunbar, Chenhall, & Bailie, 2007). Housing disadvantages can be measured and are expressed in different ways. For example, homelessness is often noted as being an extreme housing disadvantage, whereas substandard housing and the quality of a house are more moderate concerns. The gradient of housing disadvantages suffered by Aboriginal peoples will be discussed in this section.

Homelessness among Aboriginal peoples in Canada

Homelessness can be describe either by severity or duration. Using the poverty terminology, homelessness has been characterized according to its extremity: absolute, relative, or at-risk homelessness. Within these parameters, absolute homelessness refers to:

> People without shelter who may or may not live on the streets; some may rely on emergency shelters, transitional housing, friends and families. It also includes "couch surfers. These are people without shelter that sleep in different homes whenever they can (Helin, 2002).

Relative homelessness refers to the circumstances where people have a physical shelter, but the shelter does not meet basic health and safety measures (Hwang, 2001). Those at-risk of homelessness are those who are socioeconomically disadvantaged and are struggling to pay rent (Helin, 2002). The working poor is a prime example of such a group, as they continually "live on a precipice that can tumble them into homelessness at any time" (Plumb, 2000). The labelling of homelessness as "situational (or temporary) homelessness; episodic homelessness; and chronic (long-term)" (Beavis, Klos, Carter, & Douchant, 1997) has also been used. While different from the lexicon of terms used in the poverty literature, this categorization seems more intuitive, describing a dynamic continuum rather than some of the absolute and relative terms.

The literature demonstrates that homelessness is experienced by Indigenous populations around the world, although it is does not occur equally across all Indigenous populations. Some indigenous populations that disproportionately suffer from homelessness include: Native American veterans, Indigenous peoples living in the Northern Territory of Australia, and Aboriginal peoples in large cities across Canada (Carson, et al., 2007; Hwang, 2001; Kasprow & Rosenheck, 1998) but more work is needed to better understand Aboriginal homelessness. While it has been documented in the literature that patterns of migration have led to an increase in the number of urban Aboriginal people and Aboriginal homeless,, consider the following quote:

> *Increasing patterns of migration among Aboriginal people from the reserve to urban centres has led to a dramatic increase in the number of Aboriginal people now permanently residing in urban areas. Anecdotal and statistical evidence indicates that Aboriginal people are consistently and disproportionately represented among the homeless in most major Canadian cities and have unique cultural needs. No one can say with certainty the scope of the problem nor, can any accurate figure be quoted regarding the Aboriginal homeless population (Helin, 2002).*

In Toronto, however, the Toronto Star newspaper has reported that 25% of Toronto's homeless population are people of Aboriginal ancestry. With the knowledge that Aboriginal people make up only about 2% of Toronto's total population, the disproportionate representation of Aboriginal people in Toronto's homeless is evermore clear (Wente, 2000). Other numbers that suggest that Aboriginal people make up 15% of the homeless population still highlight the disproportionate over-representation of Aboriginal homeless people in the city. Since these numbers do not include the projected or at-risk populations, it is thought that the numbers could escalate by about 8000 people (Mayor's Homelessness Action Task Force, 1999). The general literature also shows that Aboriginal peoples are at an increased risk of becoming homeless (Helin, 2002).

As defined in the Greater Vancouver Regional District (GVRD) Aboriginal Homelessness Study 2003, an urban Aboriginal person is at-risk of becoming homeless if they: pay more than 25% of their income on housing; suffer from an acute life crisis; are at risk of losing accommodations; have a household income that is below one of Statistics Canada's LICOs; have low education levels; have been denied opportunity to access social housing; suffer from mental health issues; are hard to house; use food banks frequently; and are engaged in the sex trade (Dappleton Research Team, 2003).

Homelessness and Health

As the above section has shown, Aboriginal peoples are disproportionately represented in the overall homeless population, and are at a greater risk of becoming homeless. The implications of this for the health of Aboriginal peoples is important to consider, as the literature has shown that homeless people have higher than average levels of morbidity and mortality and often experience greater barriers to accessing safe and effective health care and health services. In fact, it has been noted that the homeless are at an unacceptably high risk for many preventable diseases, unnecessary health complications, and premature deaths (Plumb, 2000). The relationship between homelessness and health is reviewed in greater detail below.

Risks related to homelessness, such as exposure to the elements, poor nutrition, lack of support, poor access to health services, stigmatization, etc. can negatively impact the health and well-being of individuals and families living on the streets. In fact, homeless people are more likely to have chronic and severe medical conditions than the general population (Hwang, 2001). Health conditions among the homeless are often chronic because treatment and access to treatment is limited, sporadic, or inaccessible. Disease severity is also enhanced by the living conditions and circumstances related to homelessness. Some of the most commonly cited health problems among the homeless are: seizures, chronic obstructive pulmonary diseases, and musculoskeletal conditions (Hwang, 2001). Statistics from survey by Street Health comparing the prevalence of several chronic diseases included in this book to the non-Aboriginal population demonstrates the high risks that Aboriginal homeless people face for developing chronic conditions.

Table 1. Chronic Disease Prevalence in the Aboriginal population versus the non-Aboriginal population

Disease	Homeless Aboriginal people	Non-Aboriginal Population*
Arthritis or Rheumatism	43%	14%
Heart disease	35%	4%
Chronic Obstructive Pulmonary Disease (COPD)	24%	1%
Asthma	22%	6%
Diabetes	22%	4%

Source: (Street Health).

Note: Data for the non-Aboriginal population was drawn from the Canadian Community Health Survey (CCHS) Cycle 3.1 (2005). This analysis is based on Statistics Canada's Canadian Community Health Survey, Cycle 3.1 (2005), Public Use Microdata File, which contains anonymized data. Street Health prepared all computations on these microdata and the responsibility for the use and interpretation of these data is entirely that of the author.

In addition to these more common chronic diseases, homelessness is often thought to be related to the development and persistence of mental health conditions. While not always discussed or measured in terms of their chronic or long-term nature, mental health issues among the homeless are important. Research done in non-Indigenous populations, demonstrate that individuals with chronic mental illnesses are at greater risk for homelessness than individuals without (Folsom, et al., 2005). The table below demonstrates the high prevalence of some common mental health conditions among Aboriginal homeless people.

Table 2. Most common mental health diagnoses reported by Aboriginal people who are homeless

Mental Health Diagnosis	%
Depression	16%
Anxiety	11%
Addiction to drugs/alcohol	11%
Bipolar (manic depressive)	7%
Post traumatic stress disorder	6%
Panic disorder	6%
Schizophrenia	0%

Source: (Street Health).

Despite the truth of this and the correlation between Aboriginal and non-Aboriginal people's mental health concerns, some differences between the two groups suggests that more research is needed in this area. For example, Native American homeless veterans experienced fewer psychiatric problems and significantly more alcohol-related problems than non-Native homeless veterans (Kasprow & Rosenheck, 1998). Overall, unfortunately, Aboriginal people who are homeless report alarmingly high levels of social isolation and extremely low levels of social support. Drugs and alcohol are often used to help people cope with illness, trauma, or pain, and to relieve isolation. Given the harsh daily realities of homelessness and the legacy of historical violence and exclusion that some Aboriginal peoples in Canada endure, the high levels substance use and self-medication reported by Aboriginal people who are homeless are likely one means of coping when other options are not available. As reported by Street Health, Aboriginal people who are homeless have high levels of substance abuse. For example, the 2007 survey reported that: 92% smoke cigarettes and, of those, 89% smoke daily; 77% used an illicit drug other than marijuana regularly in the past year; 26% had injected drugs in the past year; 29% had at five or more drinks on one more occasion at least once a week in the past year; and, 15% had consumed non-beverage alcohol in the past year.[1]

In addition to the high prevalence of chronic diseases, both physical and mental, among Aboriginal homeless people, chronic diseases are often left undetected for years and are poorly controlled. Both of these situations can lead to premature mortality and excess morbidity (Hwang, 2001; Hwang & Bugeja, 2000). For instance, diabetics noted great difficulties with managing their diet and dealing with scheduling and logistics associated with personal care (Hwang & Bugeja, 2000; Plumb, 2000). Further, the Aboriginal homeless population in British Columbia (BC) has a death rate that is 2.1 times higher than the rest of BC (Helin, 2002). Concerns with the health of homeless people are also evident in their use of the health care system. Homeless people are admitted to hospitals five times more than the general population, often through emergency rooms, and stay in hospital more often than other lower-income patients (Hwang, 2001). Not only do these frequent and prolonged stays in hospitals result in high health care costs, but they also make for short-term patchwork health care that does not facilitate preventative and comprehensive health care treatment.

Substandard Housing

Poor housing conditions, overcrowding, inadequate housing supply, and lack of property ownership are prevalent in many Aboriginal communities. For these reasons and others, housing in Aboriginal communities are often substandard. A review of these housing issues and their impact on health is provided below to better understand the connection between housing and Aboriginal health in Canada.

The type of housing in First Nations communities varies, but a large proportion of on-reserve housing is old and/or in need of upgrading and

1 Non-beverage alcohol is alcohol in a form that is not meant to be consumed and includes things like mouthwash, hand sanitizer, cooking wine, and rubbing alcohol.

better maintenance. According to the 2002/03 RHS, one-third (33.6%) of First Nation homes are in need of major repairs. Another third (31.7%) need minor repairs. While the presence of household incomes below the $20,000/year cut-off were more likely to require repair and more regular maintenance, rates varied with income brackets and were still considerable high (26.4%) in more moderate income brackets ($50,000 to 79,999/year). These figures suggest systemic and underlying concerns with housing across all sectors of Aboriginal society. The fact that statistics documenting the number of houses in need of repairs have significantly increased since those reported by the 1985 Neilson Task Force is concerning for the future, as is slow progress of housing improvements noted by the 2002/03 RHS survey participants (First Nations Centre, 2005). In addition to concerns with housing construction and maintenance are concerns about the supply of housing. In 2001, Indian and Northern Affairs Canada (INAC) reported a shortage of 8,500 units on reserves (Government of Canada, 2003). The Assembly of First Nations estimates, however, that there are 80,000 backlog units (First Nations Centre, 2005). The potential impact that this housing profile may have on health is exemplified by their potential to create the conditions for mould growth, poor indoor air quality, and poor ventilation. Not surprisingly, these health concerns tend to aggravate the respiratory system, reduce lung function and growth, and lead to chronic respiratory problems (Anto, Vermeire, Vestbo, & Sunyer, 2001; Cardinal, Schopflocher, Svenson, Morrison, & Laing, 2004).

Mould can live and grow on and within the structures of the home. It has been found that moulds can produce allergies, asthma, eye and throat irritation, otitis media, and other upper and lower respiratory tract conditions (Daigler, Markello, & Cummings, 1991; First Nations Centre, 2005; J. D. O'Neil, 2000), but it is not clear how these interactions actually occur and whether there is a direct relationship between mould and specific respiratory conditions (First Nations Centre, 2005). Research has concluded, however, that a focus on mould problems does have the potential to help improve acute and chronic health conditions in communities where mould is found to be prevalent (J. D. O'Neil, 2001). As mould requires moisture to grow and thrive and about half of First Nations homes are in need of repair, the potential for a large prevalence of mould in Aboriginal homes is very real. Further, the less the ventilation, the greater the potential for mould growth. While there are measures to ensue evacuation of homes with overactive mould growth or with contamination levels that exceed the standard levels, these measures and controls are not present on reserves. This is largely due to the fact that there are few health authorities in First Nations communities with the skills and resources to do this and the lack of alternative accommodations available to send people from unfit homes to (First Nations Centre, 2005).

Issues related mould and ventilation affect the overall air quality of homes. While outdoor air quality has received a lot of media attention in the past two decades (see section 2.2.3), the potentially harmful effects of indoor air pollution is often overlooked. Such pollution is common in Aboriginal communities, where wood and coal burning stoves are still used, where tobacco is used for ceremonies and meetings, and where mould and poor ventilation are prevalent. The presence of these factors causes concern for the health and well-being of Aboriginal peoples in their homes. Through evidence of home and workplace exposures to tobacco smoke, Greer and colleagues (1993) demonstrated that indoor environments have a stronger effect on the development of respiratory problems than do outdoor air pollutants. In addition to tobacco smoke, research has shown that indoor air quality may increase the prevalence of allergies and asthma (Canadian Institute for Health Information, Canadian Lung Association, Health Canada, & Statistics Canada, 2001). The prevalence and incidence of tuberculosis and other respiratory conditions has been equated with indoor air quality (N. Bruce, Perez-Padilla, & Albalak, 2000; Hu & Ran, 2009). Since tobacco smoke and mould are the only consistent indoor factors associated with chronic conditions, more research into the influence of indoor air pollution and its various components deserve greater attention from the research community.

The potential influence of indoor air pollution on health in the future is evidenced by studies that show that Aboriginal people are spending more of their time indoors (First Nations Centre, 2005). The particular impact that indoor air pollution has on some of the most vulnerable subsets of the Aboriginal population, such as the elderly, young children and the chronically ill (who also tend to spend even more time indoors than the average individual) will also be important issues to consider.

In order to conclude this discussion about air quality, it is important to note that indoor and outdoor air quality (see section 2.2.3) are often discussed separately. While such a distinction is important to consider, it is also important to acknowledge the connection between the two: "the average house offers little protection against aerosol, particulate, and gas contamination in the general air" (First Nations Centre, 2005); poor housing offers even less. While some Aboriginal communities have reported concerns with outdoor air quality as a result of location near industrial sites, the fact that many reserves are located in rural and remote areas means that concerns related to air pollution are potentially less prominent. This means, however, that home contamination may be a greater concern for Aboriginal communities, families, and individuals (First Nations Centre, 2005).

In addition to the impact that air quality issues resulting from poor housing structure, ventilation, indoor air pollutants, and outdoor particulates have on health; crowding has also been found to aggravate the respiratory system, encourage respiratory disease transmission, and facilitate the development of chronic conditions. Unfortunately, issues of occupant density (i.e. overcrowding) have been reported in Aboriginal communities (First Nations Centre, 2005). In general, a house is considered to be overcrowded if the density exceeds one person per room (i.e. room density > 1.0). The overall room density in Canada, as reported by the 2001 Census is 0.4 persons per room, whereas the RHS reported an average density rate of 0.76 (First Nations Centre, 2005). This translates to an average of about 2.6 people per house in the non-First Nations population and 4.8 people per house in First Nations on-reserve homes. In some cases, occupancy in First Nations communities was extremely high; the highest number of people per house reported by the RHS was 18 (First Nations Centre, 2005). While statistics vary in the proportion of Aboriginal homes that are overcrowded (from 12% to 17.2%) (First Nations Centre, 2005; Indian and Northern Affairs, 2005), it is certain that homes in Aboriginal communities, on average, have more people per room than the Canadian population (First Nations Centre, 2005; Health Canada, 2002). Because research has also shown that this high proportion of overcrowding impacts an individual's and community's health and well-being, household crowding is a significant concern. For instance, it has been documented and recognized that night-time crowding is a significant risk factor for both upper and lower respiratory tract infections within the Inuit population in Greenland (Koch, et al., 2003); other studies in Aboriginal communities have also shown that overcrowding and respiratory distress are related (Fraser-Lee & Hessel, 1994). Statistics from the 2002/03 RHS report that 1 in 3 of all respondents once diagnosed with tuberculosis live in an overcrowded house. Concern for the long-term impacts of crowding on health is evidenced by the fact that 24.6% of homes with children surveyed for the 2002/03 RHS were overcrowded (First Nations Centre, 2005).

Home ownership and renting patterns are also important factors to consider when examining housing conditions among Aboriginal peoples. Differences between Aboriginal and non-Aboriginal housing is clear when comparing ownership, renting, and social housing. It has been reported from the 2001 Census that in the non-Aboriginal population, 65% of families own their home; the majority of the remainder rent, while few rely on social housing. In the First Nations population the situation is reversed: "61.9% of on-reserve families live in band-owned housing which is analogous to social housing". Comparatively, 74.1% of First Nations households on-reserve with an annual income below $10,000 and 64.4% with incomes below $30,000 live in band housing. Unusually high levels of households with annual incomes from $30,000-80,000 (57.2% for households within this range and 39.5% of the few reporting incomes above this) also report living in band-owned homes (First Nations Centre, 2005). The high occupancy of band-owned housing may be a result of poverty, banks not giving mortgages to on-reserve residents, and some geographic concerns that hinder construction access and cost. A concern with band-owned housing for the health of First Nations communities is the high percentage of mould and mildew reported (48.7%). Reports of 36.9% in other types of First Nations is also concerning (First Nations Centre, 2005). Because the urban population tends to rent more than the non-First Nations population, similar issues with mould and potential concerns with air quality and structural issues are issues of concern (Beavis, et al., 1997). As such, concerns with poor air quality and mould are equally true in these circumstances.

The close connection between one's environment and their socioeconomic situation reasserts the need to involve broader socio-cultural issues and to account for changes in air quality over time. As Aboriginal communities continue to report evidence of poor air quality, poor housing conditions, indoor air pollution, crowding, and poverty, targeted research is urgently needed to investigate the impact that these factors have on Aboriginal health and their relationship to chronic respiratory disease. Improvements seen in Aboriginal communities after relocation to better living arrangements and healthier environments substantiates (but does not causally prove) an association between respiratory health and the environment (Lawrence & Martin, 2001). A life course perspective has the potential to make this area of study more comprehensive and effective.

2.2 Geographic Risk Factors

In addition to the economic status and housing conditions of Aboriginal peoples, geographic location can exacerbate overall health and well-being by reducing access to facilities, supplies, and support services. The quality and nature of the land can also determine the health of a population. These aspects are discussed below.

2.2.1 Community Location

The geographic location of a community can be a key indicator of the health and well-being of a community. In order to investigate the relationship between location and health, regions are often classified according to their population density; proximity to an urban centre, amenities, and/or other communities; and the accessibility of the community. Some common terms include urban, suburban, rural, remote, and isolated. Directional terms are also used: mainly north and south in terms of density and accessibility differences, but also east and west in terms of land and cultural differences. As demonstrated by the figure below the Aboriginal population of Canada is situated in every province and territory, and makes up the majority of the population in Nunavut and the Northwest Territories, and is a large portion of the population in the Prairie Provinces.

Figure 2. Population reporting Aboriginal identity according to their percentage of the total population, Canada, provinces and territories, 2001

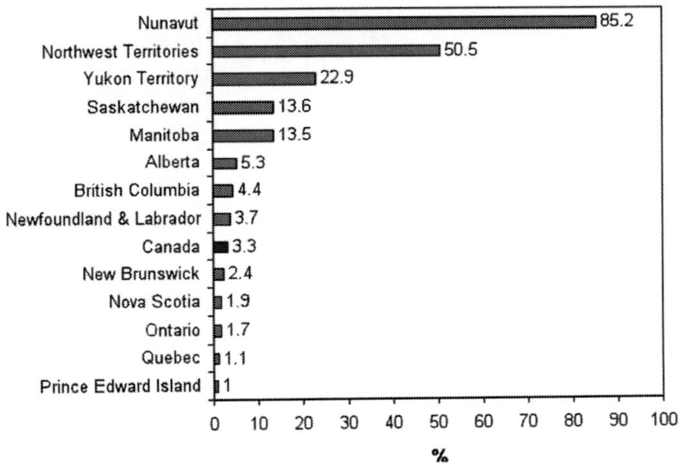

Source: (Statistics Canada, 2001b).

While this figure can be misleading – it does not provide the absolute population numbers – it does demonstrate the significance of the North for many Aboriginal peoples and the higher proportion of Aboriginal people in the more traditionally rural provinces of Saskatchewan, Manitoba, and Alberta. The term "rural" it is often used to refer a community or personal residence that is far from a large urban centre, amenities, and/or other communities. It is also used to refer to communities and locales that are only accessible in certain seasons (i.e. ice road communities), by air, or by gravel or unkempt roads. Since this is a reality for many Aboriginal peoples in Canada, the health impacts of this situation are important to review.

Regardless of ethnicity, rural location has been found to be associated with poor nutrition, inactivity, and high smoking rates. These risk factors are generally higher among the average rural population than they are among their urban counterparts (Canadian Institute for Health Information, 2006). Rural residence, particularly if it is coupled with socioeconomic risk factors, can also decrease health care access (see section 2.2.2 below for more details). Despite these negative statistics, rural and remote residency has been shown to be beneficial to the health and well-being of Aboriginal peoples. This is particularly true when rural living is equated with Northern living. This is because studies have shown that Aboriginal Northerners report lower levels of chronic diseases than other territorial residents. Further, the off-reserve Aboriginal population living in the territories was found to have a lower prevalence of chronic diseases than their provincial counterparts. This pattern seems to indicate that Aboriginal peoples living in the North may not have been exposed to the same lifestyle changes, or have experienced them to the same degree, as Southern Aboriginal communities (Tjepkema, 2002). Contradiction in the evidence can be explained by the fact that there are trade-offs between the accessibility of a community and the isolation of the community; namely, the potential negative impacts of colonization versus accessibility to amenities. Similarly one could postulate the positive benefits of more isolated and self-sufficient communities versus the impact of isolation on the diversity of community economic development opportunities.

In addition to the different environments experienced by Aboriginal peoples living in rural and Northern communities versus urban or suburban, a difference exists between on-reserve and off-reserve living. Increasingly Aboriginal peoples move to the cities with approximately 30% of Aboriginal population in Canada living on reserve (CBC News, 2003). Reserve settings have been shown to have a particular impact on health.

Social theorists have postulated that control over factors affecting one's life circumstances is associated with health. Thus, self determination has emerged as an important goal for community leaders who historically have been under the colonial control of the Federal Government. A relationship has been shown to exist between governance and health, where self-government support healthy environments and lack of control over governance issues have been equated with unhealthy behaviours and an unhealthy environment (Chandler & Lalonde, 1998). On-reserve residents have been found to have greater health risks. For instance, residents of reserves have higher mortality and morbidity rates, higher unemployment and poverty rates, and a lack of availability or access to health information and health services. Reserve residents also tend to report higher rates of some chronic diseases, such as diabetes and chronic respiratory tract infections, and higher rates of mental health problems, and drug and alcohol abuse issues (Canadian Institute for Health Information, 2006). However, Chandler and Lalonde demonstrated considerable variation among FN communities in BC above and below provincial mainstream statistical averages for suicide.

As this brief discussion demonstrates, Aboriginal peoples living on-reserve, in the Northern territories, or in other remote regions of the country are exposed to the complex of risk factors associated with their geographic location. In both reserve living and rural or Northern living, access to services is a key concern. Literature examining the impact of access issues is discussed in detail below.

2.2.2 Access to Quality Health Care

As noted in the above two sections, a community's access to health care and other health services is an important dimension of its health profile. In this case, access to quality health care refers to the availability of "Western" primary health care provisions. While access to the Western bio-medical system is important, it is also important to remember that some Aboriginal people may utilize these services in tandem with traditional health practices, only in certain context, or only for particular reasons (First Nations Centre, 2005). Issues of access are important when examining the health of populations because it has been reported in the literature that countries with better primary health care access are less likely to report health inequities (Mackinko, Starfield, & Shi, 2003). It is also important because the research shows that insufficient health care access and performance services can contribute to lower survival rates and higher mortality rates in certain populations. Given that the Aboriginal population in Canada has experienced profound health inequities compared to the non-Aboriginal population, access to services and care is a key determinant of health to investigate within this population.

The 2002/03 RHS provides some information of health care access. For instance, participants in the survey were asked to rate their health and health care access. First Nations people who rated their health as 'very good' or 'excellent' were more likely to rate their access to health services as being 'better' or the 'same' as other Canadians (24.6% and 45.5% respectively) than those who rated their health as 'good', 'fair', or 'poor'. However, actual access to health services was not significantly related to self-reported health status. Differences were also not found to be significant between the genders and across different age groups. Respondents with higher education, however, were more likely to rate their access to services lower than that of the general Canadian population (First Nations Centre, 2005).

Data from the Canadian Community Health Survey (CCHS) and the Aboriginal Peoples Survey (APS) also provide some interesting figures on the health care access of the off-reserve and on-reserve populations of Canada. For instance, data from the 2000/01 survey reported that 78.8% of Aboriginal peoples living off-reserve has seen a general practitioner at least once in the last year. Although this rate is significantly different from the non-Aboriginal population, there is an even larger difference between Aboriginal and non-Aboriginal peoples living in the Canadian territories (55.8% versus 75.9% respectively) (Tjepkema, 2002) rates of contact with general practitioners among the off-reserve Aboriginal population. The survey stated that the low rates of Northern Aboriginal peoples' contact with a regular doctor were more evident when compared with non-Aboriginal Northerners: 31.1% of off-reserve Aboriginals had a regular doctor versus 67.0% of non-Aboriginal Northern residents. While less provincially based Aboriginal people also reported having a regular doctor as well, the difference between the Aboriginal and non-Aboriginal population in the provinces was less. Interestingly, "[c]ontact with nurses were somewhat higher for Aboriginal people living in the provinces and much higher for those living in the territories" (Tjepkema, 2002). This is likely the result of the smaller community model, where community health centres are largely run and staffed by nurses. Taking into account these differences and discrepancies, it is not surprising that Tjepkema (2002) found that the off-reserve Aboriginal population cited more unmet health needs than the non-Aboriginal population. Similar results were found for the on-reserve population. The Aboriginal Peoples' Health Survey 2001 revealed that Aboriginal people residing on-reserve were "less likely to have seen a physician" or other health professional (68%) in the past year (61%) compared with the urban population (73% and 77% respectively). In addition, the proportion of Inuit who have seen a physician (47%) or other health professional (57%) in the past year was found to be the lowest among all Canadians (Newbold, 1998).

A number of barriers have been cited with regards to the accessibility of health services to the Aboriginal population. While some of the concerns vary depending on an individual's or community's location, others are broader reaching. For on-reserve, Northern and rural areas the lack of local services, lack of access to a physician or other health provider, the need to travel to get to a health facility and receive medical treatment are often cited as major barriers to adequate health care (First Nations Centre, 2005). Similarly, but more broad-reaching, are economic concerns related to issues of transportation, child care, and the direct costs of some health services. Cultural barriers, such as the lack of culturally appropriate or relevant care and issues with accessing traditional care, are also commonly cited. Finally, systemic issues include: denied approval of service under the non-Insured Health Benefits (NIHB) system or not having NIHB coverage, and long wait times for services that continue to plague many Aboriginal people, families, and communities (First Nations Centre, 2005). Seeing that the purpose of the NIHB is to help First Nations reach an overall health status similar to the non-First Nations population of Canada, data such as this suggests that the NIHB program needs to improve access to care, that this issue is a serious concern that should be addressed.

The need for local and culturally appropriate services are an important concern in the discussion of barriers to timely and appropriate access for Aboriginal peoples. Evidentiary support for this is available in the reports of better health access among individuals residing in communities with a health transfer agreement[2] (First Nations Centre, 2005). The rationale that health transfer policy enables more community control and, therefore, more culturally appropriate, culturally relevant health, and locally available services is not universally agreed to by First Nations. Interestingly, "respondents from communities that transferred as part of a multi-community transfer are more likely to rate their access to health services as generally less than Canadians" (First Nations Centre, 2005). This finding suggests the effectiveness of the health transfer system could be improved and that further research is required to assess this policy and the implications that it has on health access, health status, and general well-being.

Diagnostic, Screening, and Prevention Services

The availability of diagnostic, screening, and prevention services are often seen as indicators of health care access and performance. As such, the availability of these services in Aboriginal communities will be discussed below.

In the area of cancer, diagnostic, screening, and prevention services are thought to have a great influence on incidence, mortality and survival rates. Knowing this, the fact that the participation of members of the Aboriginal population in cancer screening programs remains lower than that of non-Aboriginal population is a concern (Young, Kliewer, Blanchard, & Mayer, 2000). Screening for cervical cancer in First Nations women through a Pap smear test has traditionally been reported as being low (Clarke, et al., 1998). Data from the 2002/03 RHS, however, shows that the level of coverage of Pap smear testing is relatively similar between the Aboriginal and non-Aboriginal populations. While this is a great improvement, the RHS states that: "given the disproportionate mortality rate First Nations women experiences as a result of cervical cancer, it would be advisable to strive for more systematic First Nations-specific screening programs" (First Nations Centre, 2005). Other research has found that in addition to issues related to access to cancer screening programs, lack of awareness of available programs and services contributes to issues related to cancer screening (Condon, Barnes, Armstrong, Selva-Nayagam, & Elwood, 2005). Thus, education and awareness should be considered an integral part of strategies to improve screening programs. Other issues related with the low uptake of

---

2 The health transfer policy was officially adopted by Health Canada in 1989 and continues today. It enables First Nations communities to control the allocation of resources for particular programs and services, thus, providing opportunity for greater autonomy and community control over health care.

certain cancer screening tests, such as the digital rectal exam require further examination (First Nations Centre, 2005).

In addition to cancer, a lack of or delayed blood sugar testing among Aboriginal peoples is thought to be connected to the rise in diabetes mellitus in this population. The 2002/03 RHS noted that less than 50% of at risk age groups had been screened for diabetes in the last 12 months (First Nations Centre, 2005). Given the epidemic proportions of diabetes in the Aboriginal population today, these numbers are far too low. Testing for cardiovascular diseases, such as cholesterol tests and blood pressure exams are also lower than is desired: cholesterol testing is low across all age groups, while blood pressure tests are being accessed at higher, but not ideal, rates (First Nations Centre, 2005). While it has been noted that, overall, screening does not generally improve or worsen in transfer communities – mostly because these communities are often in non-isolated areas – the fact that screening may be done through general practitioners and in off-reserve settings is worthy of further exploration, as certain communities may be disadvantaged by such an arrangement.

2.2.3 Climate Change, Outdoor Air Quality, and Environmental Contaminants

The importance of the environment on health has received increased attention in recent years as a result of greater public awareness and debate about the issues surrounding climate change. Because Indigenous societies are traditionally very connected to the land, issues related to climate change are amplified and/or more evident in Aboriginal contexts (Paci, Dickson, Nickels, & Furgal, 2004). The location of many Aboriginal communities in Northern and remote regions, where changes such as melting ice are much more visible than changes occurring in the Southern regions of Canada, also make the impacts more obvious.

Outdoor air quality concerns are central to discussions about climate change and the connection between the environment and human health. In response to a rising public concern for "new pollutants"[3] in the 1980's, research related to environmental conditions has focused on the presumed association between an increase in hazardous particles in the air and incidences of respiratory problems (Strachan, 2000). This hypothesis has been

3 The term, "new pollutants" is used to refer to hazardous particles and gasses (i.e. greenhouse gases) from vehicle emissions, industrial processes, and commercial practices.

corroborated by studies of non-smoking cohorts (Abbey, et al., 1995; Greer, et al., 1993), which have found significantly higher incidences of asthma and chronic respiratory symptoms among people with high cumulative exposures to particulates and ozone. The considerable influence of outdoor pollutants on human health and its potential as a risk factor for chronic respiratory disease, however, should not overshadow the potential role that indoor air pollution plays in an individual's respiratory health (Anto, et al., 2001).

Environmental concern with contaminants and the impact of industrial bi-products, chemicals, and other particulates on human health are connected to discussions of the impact of air pollution. A key concern for many First Nations and Inuit communities is exposure to polychlorinated biphenyl (PCB): they are suspected as being responsible for increased cancer incidence rates and other health issues. PCBs accumulate in tissues bioconcentrate up the food chain, and Aboriginal people who consume fish and sea mammals as a signifigant part of their traditional diet have been found to have a very high concentration of PCBs in their body fat. A recent Canadian study found that Inuit women living in Northern Quebec have seven times the PCB concentration in their milk than that of other Canadian women (MacMillan, MacMillan, Offord, & Dingle, 1996). Moreover, the breast milk of these Aboriginal women was found to have the highest PCB concentration in the world. At the same time, the Government of Canada has reported that the PCB concentration required to cause cancer is far greater than any possible environmental exposure (Health Canada, 1994; Murray, 1994). Mercury accumulated in fish tissues is another reason for concern for many Aboriginal communities, especially those that rely on fish as a primary food source (Van Oostdam, et al., 2005). Inorganic and methyl mercury have been designated probable carcinogens; this means that at high levels they can increase cancer risk. According to a study involving Inuit living in a Baffin Island community, their daily intake of mercury averaged 65 mg for women and 97 mg for men, which is much higher than the mean daily intake of 16 mg for mainstream Canadians (MacMillan, et al., 1996). Since mercury has been linked to other health conditions, such as nervous system problems and learning disabilities, this is a key concern for the future health and well-being of Aboriginal Peoples.

The risk of eating traditional foods need to recognize the competing risk of store bought alternatives which are often costly, low in nutrients and high in fat, salt and sugar. The challenge of environmental contaminants in the food chain is that they are often found in "traditional" or "country" foods; the general category used to describe all of organic plant and animal nutrients that ensure and maintain the health of Aboriginal Peoples (Paci, et al., 2004). In Canada, common country/traditional foods are fish, wild game, berries, and other gathered vegetables, fruits, and grains. The importance of discussing the past, present, and future gathering and consumption of traditional/country foods among Aboriginal Peoples in Canada is that they can be protective factors for many chronic diseases. The correlation between the consumption of country foods and better health is also a result of the higher nutrient value of these foods and the traditional physical activity associated with the hunting and gathering required to obtain them. While these modern or western foods have been assimilated into Indigenous communities at different times, speeds, and intensities (Paci, et al., 2004), their presence is now common and widespread. In addition to encouraging the reduction of traditional foods in Indigenous diets, these cheap and easy access foods are often unhealthy. Carbonated sugar drinks, salted and fried potato chips, and other "empty-calorie" foods do not provide the nutrients, vitamins, and minerals that are needed to survive and thrive.

The effects of greenhouse gas emissions and society's carbon footprint on the land and the health of people, the costs and concerns with the fuel and logistics of the transportation of food to rural and remote communities, are another reason for encouraging the harvesting and consumption of country foods. Thus, it will be imperative to find more innovative ways to ensure a balance between food availability, diversity, and quality.

3. Prenatal Risk Factors

The term "prenatal risk factors" is used here to denote those that occur, exist, or act on the individual prior to birth. As such, prenatal risk factors are associated with the health of the mother. Included in this section, therefore, is a discussion of maternal diabetes, maternal obesity, maternal smoking, and maternal alcohol use. While birth weight is often an indicator of intrauterine effects, birth weight will be explicitly discussed in the natal risk factor section, which follows this section. It was placed in the natal section, as it is measure at the time of birth and impacts the infant's health and its chronic disease risk.

3.1 Maternal Diabetes

As noted in the next chapter (see Part III, section 2, sub-section 2.2.2 for more details), First Nations women represent roughly two-thirds of the First Nations people who are diagnosed with diabetes (Bobet, 1997), while the reverse is true in the general Canadian population (Health Canada, 1999). In addition to experiencing an overall higher prevalence of type 2 diabetes (First Nations Centre, 2005), many First Nations women are also diagnosed with gestational diabetes mellitus (GDM) (Mohamed & Dooley, 1998), which is defined as any degree of glucose intolerance for which the onset or first recognition occurred during pregnancy (Matthews, 2003). This section is intended to review the impact that high rates of GDM in Aboriginal mothers have on the fetus and, therefore, the future generations.

Research shows that GDM is a strong predictor of high birth weight in newborns (Dyck, Klomp, & Tan, 2001; Godwin, Muirhead, Huynh, Helt, & Grimmer, 1999; Harris, Caulfield, Sugamori, Whalen, & Henning, 1997; Rodrigues, Robinson, & Gray-Donald, 1999). In addition to increased rates of macrosomia (high birth weight > 4.0 kg), offspring of women with GDM may also experience increased impaired glucose tolerance (IGT), increased rates of childhood obesity, and an increased risk of type 2 diabetes (Damm, 2009; Pettitt, 1998; Silverman, Rizzo, Cho, & Metzger, 1998). A study of Pima Indians indicated a significant association of maternal glucose intolerance with elevated risk of diabetes in offspring (Franks, et al., 2006). Since GDM and high birth weight are also linked, the question is whether it is the high birth weight or the mother's diabetes that increases the risk to the health of Aboriginal children. However, a study among Pima Indians, which examined families where siblings were born both before and after their mother was diagnosed with diabetes, demonstrated that children exposed to diabetes in utero had a higher body mass index (BMI) than their unexposed siblings and that their risk of diabetes was almost four times higher (Dabelea, et al., 2000). In another study, it was suggested that about 40% of type 2 diabetes among 5- to 19-year-old Pima children can be attributed to GDM during pregnancy (Dabelea & Pettitt, 2001). This discussion of maternal diabetes highlights the potentially strong impact that the fetal environment plays an individual's health later in life.

3.2 Maternal Obesity

Some studies suggest that maternal obesity, which is often associated with GDM, may be the overriding factor in mediating offspring obesity (Boney, Verma, Tucker, & Vohr, 2005; Whitaker, Pepe, Seidel, Wright, & Knopp, 1998). An American study that followed children from birth to 6-12 years found that GDM was not independently significant in increasing metabolic syndrome[4] risk in children, but offspring of obese mothers incurred a two-fold increased risk profile (Boney, Verma, Tucker, & Vohr, 2005). If these results could be extended to Canada's Aboriginal population, pre-pregnancy and pregnancy could be seen as an extremely effective point in the life course to target obesity and thus reduce the burden of type 2 diabetes throughout the early years and adulthood. In general, these results also demonstrate the strong relationship between maternal health and the health of a child at birth and throughout their life. The literature on the impact of another maternal lifestyle behaviour, smoking, on fetal development and chronic disease risk is discussed below.

3.3 Maternal Smoking

A clear association has been shown between maternal smoking and intrauterine growth restriction in both Aboriginal and non-Aboriginal populations (Horta, Victora, Menezes, Halpern, & Barros, 1997; Power & Jefferis, 2002; Wenman, Joffres, & Tataryn, 2004). The proportion of pregnant women who smoke varies substantially among different ethnic groups. According to RHS 2002-2003, smoking rates among pregnant First Nation women (58.8%) matched those in the general First Nations population (First Nations Centre, 2005). When compared to the Canadian average, however, maternal smoking rates are almost twice as high (36.6% vs. 19.4%) (First Nations Centre, 2005). A study conducted in Manitoba found that among 684 interviewed women a significantly higher proportion of Aboriginal women (61.2%) than non-Aboriginal women (26.2%) smoked during pregnancy; however, a smaller proportion of Aboriginal women than non-Aboriginal reported smoking > one pack per day (Heaman & Chalmers, 2005). These findings are contrary to the results of the 2002/03 RHS, which found that Aboriginal mothers smoking > 10 cigarettes per day were

4 Metabolic syndrome is not a disease in and of itself, but is a cluster of disorders of an individual's metabolism — including high blood pressure, high insulin levels, excess body weight and abnormal cholesterol levels — that make them more or less likely to develop diabetes, heart disease and/or a stroke.

three times higher than mothers in the general Canadian (15.0% vs. 5.3% respectively). Perhaps this means that moderate smoking is more common among Aboriginal mothers, whereas more extreme smoking habits are more common in the non-Aboriginal population.

In both Aboriginal and non-Aboriginal populations, the mean number of cigarettes smoked by pregnant women in both populations decreased as pregnancy progressed. This and the consistently higher rates of maternal smoking in Aboriginal populations are represented in the following figure.

Figure 3. Prevalence of smoking across the stages of pregnancy for non-Aboriginal and Aboriginal pregnant women in Manitoba

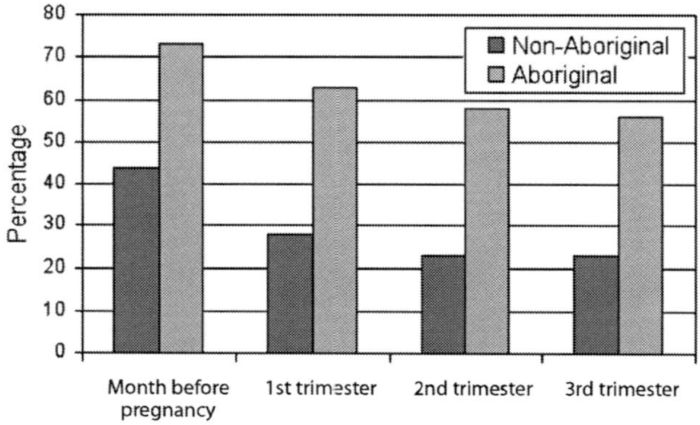

Source: (Heaman & Chalmers, 2005).

As explained by Heaman and Chalmers (2005), a number of factors influence maternal smoking habits. For example, there was a significant relationship between smoking during pregnancy for Aboriginal mothers with low-income, alcohol use during pregnancy, low support from others, inadequate prenatal care, a family history of residential school attendance, low education levels, and location in a remote and isolated community. Conversely, having a paid job and living in communities with multi-community health services reduced the odds of smoking during pregnancy (Heaman & Chalmers, 2005). In addition to active smoking by mothers in Aboriginal communities, maternal exposure to tobacco smoke is important to consider. Since statistics demonstrate that the presence of smoking in the home of First Nations mothers was about one in every two families (48.2%), passive maternal smoking can be considered an important issue. The generally high prevalence of active and passive maternal smoking in Aboriginal populations is why it is important to examine the potential impact that maternal smoking has on disease later in life (Grove, et al., 2001; Reilly, et al., 2005; von Kries, Toschke, Koletzko, & Slikker, 2002); this is reviewed below.

Negative effects of maternal smoking on fetal growth has been well-documented: numerous studies have shown that smoking tobacco during pregnancy causes fetal growth retardation (FGR) (Cliver, et al., 1995; Jackson, Batiste, & Rendall-Mkosi, 2007), which may result in low birth weight (Humphrey & Holzheimer, 2000; Mohsin, Bauman, & Jalaludin, 2005) or sometimes in preterm births (< 37 weeks), stillbirths, and neonatal deaths (Chan, Keane, & Robinson, 2001; Kallen, 2001; Mohsin, et al., 2005; Shah & Bracken, 2000). The 2002/03 RHS found that low birth weight is linked to heavy prenatal maternal smoking (when mothers smoked ≥ 20 cigarettes per day). Smoking has also been directly associated with central metabolic syndrome and has been documented as a concern for the development of chronic respiratory diseases, such as asthma in children (Daigler, et al., 1991). This is because fetal exposure to smoke can impair the proper development of the pulmonary system in utero (Gilliland, et al., 2000; Hanrahan, et al., 1992). This is why infants born to women who smoke are at the higher risk of respiratory infections and asthma compared with infants of non-smoking mothers (Gilliland, et al., 2000; Hanrahan, et al., 1992; Heaman & Chalmers, 2005). The long-term impacts of smoking among Aboriginal mothers have also been reported. According to the 2002/03 RHS, children who were exposed to smoking during their fetal gestation were less likely to report 'excellent' or 'very good' health and were more likely to have chronic bronchitis, ear infections, asthma and allergies than unexposed children. There is also a trend towards worse overall performance in infants exposed to smoking during fetal gestation (First Nations Centre, 2005). These long-term trends are particularly concerning for the future health and well-being of Aboriginal peoples.

3.4 Maternal Alcohol Use

The toxic effects of alcohol on the fetus may result in fetal alcohol effects (FAE) or fetal alcohol syndrome (FAS), depending on the amount of alcohol consumed during pregnancy. While debated, Health Canada suggests that regular consumption of 2 drinks a day or more is toxic to fetus and may lead to FAE/FAS (Canada, 2005a).

The physical, mental, emotional and behavioural effects of fetal exposure to alcohol vary widely among affected individuals. Fetal alcohol syndrome is generally characterized by distinct facial characteristics, growth retardation, and dysfunction of the central nervous system (Anderson, et al., 2002; BC FAS Resource Society, 1998; Tait, 2003; Van Bibber, 1997; Wemigwans, 2005). Fetal alcohol effects are the behavioural and cognitive effects observed in the absence of the physical malformations of FAS. This can cause complications for determining prevalence and incidence rates because many people affected by prenatal alcohol exposure do not display obvious physical symptoms, but instead will suffer from more cognitive and behavioural symptoms. Because these symptoms are more difficult to diagnose, they often remain undetected until the affected child goes to school. This means that the true incidence of FAE is likely much higher than the reported rates of FAS/FAE in newborns (Canadian Pediatric Society, 2002; Square, 1997). In addition to the terms FAS and FAE, the term fetal alcohol spectrum disorder (FASD) is used to encompass "the full range of outcomes observed among individuals with prenatal alcohol exposure" (Rasmussen, Horne, & Witol, 2006). This term will be generally used throughout this section to refer to prenatal alcohol exposure, unless a direct reference to FAS or FAE is provided.

Occurrence and severity of FASD symptoms are known to vary between affected individuals, but recent evidence suggests the presence of differences at the population level, between affected Aboriginal and non-Aboriginal children. The FASD literature does document some noticeable differences between the Aboriginal and non-Aboriginal population in Canada. For instance, it has been estimated that overall FAS incidence in the general Canadian population is between 2.8 and 4.8 per 1000 of live birth. Comparably, the rate of FAS in the Northern Manitoba Aboriginal population was 7.2 per 1000 of live births (Canadian Pediatric Society, 2002). The 2002/03 RHS found that on a national level, the prevalence rate of FASD among First Nations is 1.8% (First Nations Centre, 2005).

Comparisons made between FASD prevalence rates between Aboriginal and non-Aboriginal Canadians, however, should be regarded with caution. This is because studies of FASD among Aboriginal Peoples have typically focused on small communities believed to be at risk of fetal alcohol exposure due to high rates of binge drinking (Tait, 2003). As such, these communities tend to demonstrate extraordinarily high prevalence rates; sometimes as high as one in five births (Van Bibber, 1997). For example, a study of alcohol use by pregnant women on Vancouver Island has found that 54% of Aboriginal (Canadian Pediatric Society, 2002) and 16% of non-Aboriginal (Square, 1997) pregnant women were found to be at risk of having a newborn with some FAE. In addition to research being conducted in high-risk communities, it is often thought that a number of other factors may be influencing the high rates of FASD reported in Aboriginal communities. For example, researcher expectations of documenting such high rates; more Aboriginal than non-Aboriginal women providing accurate descriptions of alcohol use during pregnancy; a greater likelihood of health professionals diagnosing FASD in Aboriginal patients; and small groups of women consuming alcohol during multiple pregnancies (Tait, 2003).

In addition to these issues, research on FASD is skewed due to the fact that the alarmingly high FASD prevalence rates among some Aboriginal communities (or clusters of individuals) are often generalized to all Aboriginal peoples, without evidence to do so and without regard for the diversity that exists among Aboriginal peoples (Tait, 2003; Van Bibber, 1997). As more research begins to develop across the country, in both high and low risk areas, it will be possible to get a better picture of the scope of FASD. Evidence from the States documenting that prevalence rates of FASD differ between American Indian tribes based on control and structure of government (Tait, 2003) will be important to take into account, as these differences may also influence the stratification of FASD in Canada. As alcohol abuse (see section 7.2) is common in many Aboriginal communities and FASD is widely recognized as the leading cause of preventable birth defects in their children (BC FAS Resource Society, 1998; Canada, 2005b), this issue will be important to consider with regards to the long-term health of the Aboriginal population.

4. Natal Risk Factors

"From an Indigenous perspective, each new life might be considered as an opportunity from the creator for hope and healing, for individuals, families, communities, and nations. On the medicine wheel…infants sit beside the elders. Like elders, they may be considered teachers. Elders and infants are both close to the spirit world; the infants arriving from it, and the elders traveling to it. This closeness to the spirit world may bring a spiritual strength, but it may also bring a physical vulnerability and sensitivity to environmental disturbance" (First Nations Centre, 2005).

The term "natal" is generally used to refer to things relating to, associated with, or present at one's birth. Natal health is so important because a child's risk of dying is highest in the first month of life, when safe childbirth and effective neonatal care are essential (WHO, 2007). Further, children are exposed to important risk factors for the development of chronic diseases at this stage; abnormal birth weights and breastfeeding are two that will be specifically discussed here. As will be demonstrated by these factors below, the health of Aboriginal infants is interrelated with maternal, family, and community health.

4.1 Abnormal birth weights

In the world of Western medicine, birth weight is considered one of the most important measures of infant health. This is because birth weight can be used to measure fetal growth, to assess conditions in the womb, and to link these early life factors to health in adulthood (First Nations Centre, 2005). Several studies have illustrated the association between sub-optimal patterns of fetal and infant growth and adult chronic disease. These studies lay the foundation for what is known as the "*fetal origins hypothesis,*" which suggests that physiologic or metabolic "programming" during gestation and infancy determines, to a large extent, the occurrence of various chronic diseases in later life (Barker, 1995a, 1995b, 1995c; Hales & Barker, 1992). For instance, a number of studies have reported a strong link between low birth weight and the occurrence of heart disease and hypertension later in life (Barker, 1995a, 1995b, 1995c; Hales & Barker, 1992; Nair, Nair, & Chacko, 2009). Historical cohort studies in England have found that impaired fetal growth, low birth weight, and lower respiratory tract infections in early childhood are associated with lower levels of lung function in late adult life (Barker, et al., 1991; Shaheen, et al., 1994). Although a 1985-86 follow-up study was unable to confirm this finding (Shaheen, Sterne, Tucker, & Florey, 1998), Barker and colleagues (1991) added to this theory when he found an association between lower birth weights and poorer adult lung function. The biological explanation of this association is that the intrauterine influences that slow fetal weight gain also constrain the growth of the airways and permanently effect their development and function (Barker, 2004). One problem with these studies, however, is that they often assume that a higher birth weight is healthier: this assumption does not account for maternal conditions, such as obesity and diabetes, that might cause changes in the intrauterine environment that will produce heavier, but not necessarily healthier, babies (K. N. Chan, Wong, & Silverman, 1990; Coory, 2000).

For instance, both high (> 4.0 kg) and low (< 2.5 kg) birth weights have been shown to be associated with increased risk for diabetes in later life (Harder, Rodekamp, Schellong, Dudenhausen, & Plagemann, 2007; Pettitt, Forman, Hanson, Knowler, & Bennett, 1997; Pettitt & Knowler, 1998). Despite increased smoking during pregnancy among Aboriginal women, which has been shown to decrease birth weights (Pirogowicz, et al., 2004; Wenman, Joffres, & Tataryn, 2004), Aboriginal and Canadian populations have similar proportions of births with low birth weight (Gilchrist, et al., 2004). Despite high rates of maternal smoking in Aboriginal communities, First Nations babies are almost twice as likely to be classified with a high birth weight than non-Aboriginal Canadians (Rodrigues, Robinson, Kramer, & Gray-Donald, 2000). The mean birth weight for First Nations children reported by the 2002/03 RHS was 3.55 kg and the mean weight for males (3.60 kg) was higher than it was for girls (3.49 kg). While the mean birth weight is on the higher end of the "normal birth weight" range (2.5-4.0 kg), the gender difference is not considered to be a significant finding: higher birth weight among males has been reported in non-Aboriginal populations (First Nations Centre, 2005). A major concern with high birth weight is its association with the rising epidemic of diabetes among Aboriginal peoples (Caulfield, Harris, Whalen, & Sugamori, 1998; Kaijser, et al., 2009). A recent study of First Nations births in Saskatchewan from 1950 to 1984 showed a significant association between high birth weight (but not low birth weight) and diabetes for Saskatchewan registered Indians (OR 1.63 [95% CI 1.20, 2.24]). This trend was also found to be stronger for females than males (Dyck, Klomp, & Tan, 2001). The researchers in this study suggested that excess fetal nutrition is the overriding intrauterine factor in the pathogenesis of type 2 diabetes in the Canadian Aboriginal population. As discussed earlier, the prevalence of maternal diabetes is also thought to affect birth weight. A study conducted in Saskatchewan among First Nations women found that infants from GDM pregnancies were 2.4 times more likely to be macrosomic (95% CI: 1.1, 5.6) than their non-GDM counterparts (Dyck, et al., 2001). High birth weight was also found to be a factor in the development of childhood asthma. Sin et al. (2004) concluded that "because obesity promotes inflammations and imposes mechanical constraints to the airways, a high birth weight may be a risk factor for asthma in childhood". Since Aboriginal children have been documented to have higher birth weights than non-Aboriginal children (Sin, Sharpe, Cowie, & Man, 2004; Thomson, 1990), they may be at a greater risk of developing chronic respiratory illness early in life.

Nevertheless, it is important to not over-generalize about the prevalence of high birth weight among Aboriginal children. This is because, on the one hand, studies, such as those involving the James Bay Cree have reported among the highest mean birth weight statistics and a high prevalence of infant macrosomia (Rodrigues, et al., 2000). Similarly, other studies have suggested that Aboriginal children are genetically predisposed to high birth weights (Sin, et al., 2004). However, poor fetal development and low birth weight has been documented in many disadvantaged and/or marginalized Aboriginal communities (Blair, 1996; A. Chan, Keane, & Robinson, 2001), where access to basic necessities and medical care puts mothers and their infants at risk. A prevalence of poor living conditions, socioeconomic problems, and inadequate maternal health care in many Aboriginal communities places these infants at a high risk for low birth weight (Blair, 1996; A. Chan, et al., 2001). Thus, before conclusions can be drawn about this risk factor, more research and understanding is needed (Blair, 1996; A. Chan, et al., 2001).

A final point must be made about the classification of birth weights. Currently, Aboriginal birth weights are classified as high, normal or low in comparison to non-Aboriginal standards. Because of potential differences between Aboriginal and non-Aboriginal populations in terms of maternal and child health, birth weight correlations should be considered rudimentary and preliminary at best. More appropriate and culturally specific measures of Aboriginal birth weights are needed in the future so that more accurate statistics can be used to assess this risk factor in the Aboriginal context.

4.2 Breastfeeding

Breastfeeding is a common topic in natal health. While the popularity of breastfeeding among mothers has varied with the times and continues to vary according to cultural contexts and perspectives, there is a growing body of literature discussing its impact on infant health and development.

Health Canada encourages mothers to breastfeed because it provides infants with nutritional and emotional nurturing, as well as immunological benefits that enhance an infant's growth and development (Health Canada, 2000a). Breastfeeding is considered to be an important aspect of disease prevention, because infants who are breastfed have an increased protection against respiratory, ear, and intestinal infections. This is because the unique components of human milk helps protect infants from outside infection (Health Canada, 2000a). Children who are breastfed are reported as being less likely to be overweight, more likely to be of an acceptable weight, and more likely to be in "very good" or "excellent" health. These results support literature on the perceived benefits of breastfeeding. In addition to the health benefits, breastfeeding is socially and economically advantageous, since it is an ecologically sound, efficient, economical, and self-reliant food source (Breastfeeding Committee for Canada, 2002; Health Canada, 2000).

Like all babies born prior to the advent of formula, native infants were nursed until they were able to digest other food sources (Banks, 2003). Traditional breastfeeding practices, however, shifted to bottle-feeding in the 1950s when formula was introduced to the population (MacMillan, et al., 1996). For example, a study of Native children in Manitoba identified prolonged breastfeeding as a strong protective factor against type 2 diabetes: a child who was breastfed for more than 12 months was shown to have only 24% of the risk of diabetes compared with a bottle-fed child (K. Young, Chateau, & Zhang, 2002). The protective effects of breastfeeding have also been observed in Pima Indian studies (Pettitt, et al., 1997; Pettitt & Knowler, 1998). Despite these studies and the fact that initiation rates for breastfeeding has increased in recent years (Langner & Steckle, 1991; Macaulay, Hanusaik, & Beauvais, 1991), the limited statistics documenting Aboriginal breastfeeding rates report lower breastfeeding rates than those of women in the non-Aboriginal population (Dodgson, Duckett, Garwick, & Graham, 2002).

For instance, a 1988 survey conducted for the National Database on Breastfeeding among Indian and Inuit Women revealed that 60.7% of infants were breastfed at birth, but the rate dropped dramatically to 31.1% by the time the infants were 6 months old (Langner & Steckle, 1991). A more recent study of James Bay Cree found a breastfeeding initiation rate of 51.9% among Aboriginal mothers (Black, Godwin, & Ponka, 2008). The average proportion of children reported by the RHS 2002/03 who are breastfed was 62.5% (First Nations Centre, 2005). As noted in the RHS: "This rate is higher than the previous rate (50%) reported for First Nations and Inuit (First Nations and Inuit Regional Health Survey National Steering Committee, 1999). However, it is lower than the rate (79.9%) that was reported for the general Canadian population (Statistics Canada, 1999b). The RHS also reported on the duration of breastfeeding: "of the children who were breastfed, 21.6% were breastfed for 12 weeks or less, and 35% were breastfed for three to six months and 43.3% were breastfed for more than six months" (First Nations Centre, 2005). These rates were found to be higher than the rates reported from the 1997 RHS (only 22.5% reported breastfeeding for more than seven months) (First Nations and Inuit Regional Health Survey National Steering Committee, 1999). In comparison with the Canadian population, 32.5% reported breastfeeding for 12 weeks or less, 33.4% for three to six months, and 34.0% for more than six months (Statistics Canada, 1999b).

The socio-cultural, political, and economic forces connected to breastfeeding are complex (Banks, 2003). For instance, the success or failure of breastfeeding among many Aboriginal women is connected to many intergenerational and community factors. Among Mohawk women, breastfeeding is strongly influenced by the baby's grandmother, who plays a key role in the child's rearing. Thus, breastfeeding rates are often low because it is an impractical form of feeding if grandmothers and extended family are to also be involved. Since bottle feeding makes the involvement of the extended family more possible and pump technology and storage is not always available, feeding practices tend to be different than among the non-Aboriginal population. Other cultural influences, such as the availability of government-subsidized baby formula, can encourage low breastfeeding rates (Banks, 2003). Furthermore, mothers with low income, a family history of residential school attendance, and/or living in a community that had a multi-community health services agreement were lower and shorter in duration (First Nations Centre, 2005). While this information from the 2002/03 RHS is helpful, the relationship between breastfeeding and these and other factors, such as education, need to be investigated further (Breastfeeding Committee for Canada, 2002). The association reported by the RHS between high birth weight, breastfeeding, and non-smoking mothers also deserves attention (First Nations Centre, 2005).

5. Early Childhood Risk Factors

The stage known as "early childhood" refers to children aged one to five years old. This age-range is often separated out because it is during this time that children experience a phase of accelerated growth. This time period is particularly important for health because it is this growth period that has the potential to influence one's long-term health and development: "A good foundation in the early years makes a difference through adulthood, thus, giving a better start to the next generation" (WHO, 2008a).

While the care of children during this time is often placed on the shoulders of the parents, it is increasingly recognized that it is extremely important for service providers, planners and policymakers to thoroughly understand the significance of early childhood and to play a role in ensuring the social, economic, and biological needs of all children are met (Centres of Excellence for Children's Well-being, 2008). The need to focus on this area is so important because it is sadly the first time in history that parents can confidently say that their children are likely have a lower life expectancy than themselves (Chronic Disease Prevention Alliance of Canada, 2006). In an effort to provide increased awareness about the impacts of early childhood on chronic diseases later in life, this section will review the key risk factors for chronic diseases present for Aboriginal children. First, however, a description of the population will be provided.

5.1 Population Influences

A defining feature of the Aboriginal population is its young age and high birth rate. As a result, the Aboriginal population is the fastest growing population group in Canada (its birth rate is one and a half times higher than the non-Aboriginal population) (Statistics Canada, 1996) and Aboriginal children account for a large portion of the total Aboriginal population. According to a report by the Canadian Council on Social Development (CCSD) in 2002, children under the age of 14 represent one-third of the Aboriginal population, which is considerably higher than the 19% of the population that non-Aboriginal children represent (J. Anderson, 2003). Further, statistics from 2002 show that Aboriginal children account for 5.6% of the total number of children in Canada, while the total Aboriginal population accounts for 3.3% of the total population of Canada (J. Anderson, 2003). Because of the large percentage that Aboriginal children make up of the total population and because they represent the future, their health and well-being must be considered an important area of focus. The risk factors for chronic diseases with greatest exposure and impact in childhood will be discussed here, so as to better understand the present and future health and well-being of Aboriginal children.

5.2 Child Poverty and Hunger

About 20 million children under age five worldwide are severely malnourished and live in impoverished conditions. As a result, these children are more vulnerable to illness and early death (WHO, 2008a). While the terms poverty and hunger are often equated with developing countries, the reality of child poverty in Canada is very real: one in six children in Canada is living in poverty. This makes for a child poverty rate of about 15%, three times the rates of Sweden, Norway, and Finland (ending child poverty – MPH). Poverty among Aboriginal children is even more appalling. While some of the statistics are conflicting, approximately one in four First Nations children live in poverty (Campaign 2000, 2006). However, a report from 2001 documented that more than half (52.1%) of Aboriginal children were poor (Lee, 2000).

When statistics were broken down for on- and off-reserve children, the large number of Aboriginal children in poverty is evermore clear. This is because 40% of off-reserve Aboriginal children live in poverty (Campaign 2000, 2006). And, since 219,570 of the 286,500 Aboriginal children live off-reserve, this means that "77% of all Aboriginal children between the ages of zero and nine" could be considered as living in poverty. This shockingly high statistic represents the highest rate of the three "equity groups" noted in and pictured by Figure 4 (Lee, 2000).

Figure 4. Prevalence of Child Poverty in Aboriginal, Visible Minority Children, and Children with Disabilities (0-14 years)

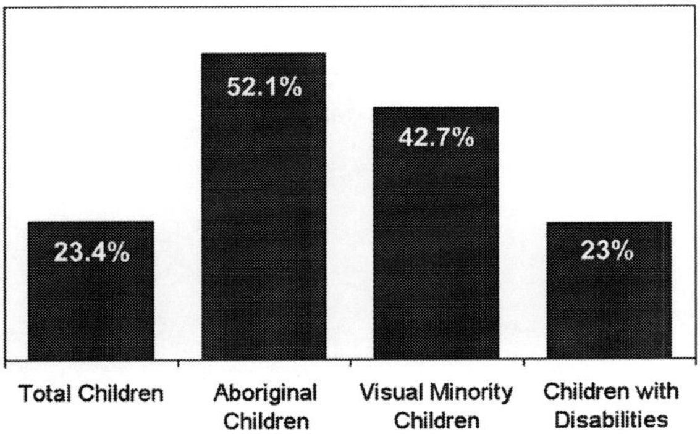

Source: (J. Anderson, 2003).

Note: In this table, Aboriginal refers to those persons who identified themselves with being North American Indian, Métis or Inuit. Visible minority persons are defined under the Employment Equity Act (1986) as those (other than Aboriginal persons) who are non-Caucasian in race or non-white in colour. Persons with disabilities are identified based on their responses to questions regarding their activity limitations or disabilities.

While the statistics on poverty among Aboriginal children are shocking, the real concern behind the numbers in the impact of this state of being on the health of Aboriginal peoples now and in the future. This is because, "[p] overty rates are indicators of the health of citizens and the state of institutes. As well, poverty rates are predictors of long-term health issues in children" (Ontario Federation of Indian Friendship Centres, 2004). No matter how you look at the numbers, then, one can conclude that the current and future health of Aboriginal children is at serious risk. The intergenerational impact of poverty and the connection between child poverty and family poverty will be discussed with regard to the particular impact of poverty on a child's health and development.

5.2.1 The impact of child poverty on adult health

It is logical to assume that an adult's socioeconomic status is associated with their socioeconomic status as a child. But since not all adults with low socioeconomic status grow up in poor socioeconomic conditions (and vice versa), understanding the patterns of socioeconomic status throughout the life course is needed to elucidate its association with an individual's health status.

It is now well accepted that childhood origins can shape adult health through material deprivation and their influence on adult circumstances and behaviour, there is increasing evidence that childhood circumstances also affect developmental health (Boyce & Keating, 2004). As has been highlighted by McEwen and colleagues, recurrent stress responses triggered in early life by adverse social environments can initiate enduring physiological changes, such as alterations in lipid metabolism and the accumulation of body fat, the development of hypertension, and the development of insulin resistance that leads to type 2 diabetes mellitus and cardiovascular disease (McEwen, 2006). Several other studies have demonstrated the link between poverty in childhood and chronic diseases later in life (Cohen & Reutter, 2007; Everson, Maty, Lynch, & Kaplan, 2002; Galobardes, Lynch, & Davey Smith, 2004; Lawlor & Smith, 2005; Poulton, et al., 2002; Power, et al., 2007). In a Norwegian study, the highest risk of mortality among men and women was observed in the group that was poor both in childhood and in adulthood; this demonstrates a clear cumulative influence of social circumstances across the life course on mortality risk (Claussen, Davey Smith, & Thelle, 2003). In the same study, cardiovascular mortality was more strongly associated with childhood than with adulthood social circumstances. Thus, the latent effects of poverty on adult health show that the gradient of health begins to emerge in childhood (Graham & Power, 2004; Moody-Ayers, Lindquist, Sen, & Covinsky, 2007; Poulton, et al., 2002). This is largely considered to be due to a number of intersecting factors including, but not limited to, poor nutrition and access to health care (Graham & Power, 2004). Further, the patterning of behaviour and lifestyle habits, which occurs in childhood, is thought to have a profound effect on future health and development.

5.2.2 Hunger and food security

Deeply connected with poverty is deprivation of nutrients and/or one's inability to access, buy, and consume an adequate amount of food with sufficient nutrients. It is not surprising, then, that the most pressing concern of Aboriginal children living in poverty is a lack of food. In fact, the Canadian Council on Social Development has found that Aboriginal children are four times more likely to be hungry than any other ethnic minority in Canada (J. Anderson, 2003; McIntyre, 2003). Understanding what this means for the health of children living in poverty requires a brief review of the meaning of malnutrition and its impact on health.

According to McIntyre (2003), "[m]alnutrition is defined as failure to achieve nutrient requirements, which can impair physical or mental health". Thus, some common effects of poverty-induced malnutrition on health are mental, while others are physical (Ontario Federation of Indian Friendship Centres, 2004). For instance, a child's ability to concentrate in school has been linked to food consumption (particularly access to breakfast). Stunted growth or low height for age, arguably the most accurate measures of malnutrition, demonstrate the more physical aspects of inadequate food consumption (McIntyre-food security, policy options). An additional concern with malnutrition is the consumption and absorption of important micronutrients, such as iron, iodine, and vitamin A (McIntyre, 2003). While the term malnutrition is a useful and effective word for describing hunger in developing countries, it has been argued that food insecurity is a better term to use when describing hunger in developed societies, such as Canada. Food insecurity is defined by McIntyre (2003) as: "the inability to acquire or consume an adequate diet quality or sufficient quantity of food in socially acceptable ways, or the uncertainty that one will be able to do so". Whether described as food insecurity or malnutrition, the ability for one to meet adequate nutritional levels consistently and completely is a key determinant of health (Ontario Federation of Indian Friendship Centres, 2004).

While the particular impacts of child hunger on long term health and development are complex and interact with the experiences of low socio-economic status that often predispose children to hunger, it is important to keep in mind that "child hunger is the extreme manifestation of household food insecurity" (McIntyre, 2003). Thus, a community perspective is useful.

5.2 Early child learning and development

In addition to physical growth and development, a critical stage for optimizing intellectual and social development occurs in the early years. This cognitive and social growth is often facilitated through family and community activities as well as participation and attendance in high quality early childhood development or preschool programs (Palacio-Quintin, 2000; Statistics Canada, 2001c). According to the 2001 Aboriginal Peoples Survey (APS), just over half (53%) of Aboriginal children aged 6 to 14 years living in non-reserve areas had attended an early childhood development program when they were younger. Inuit children were less likely to have attended a preschool program (35%) compared to First Nations (54%) and Métis (57%) children. Programs specifically designed to meet the needs of Aboriginal children, however, are increasing and these seem to have greatly increased enrolment and retention rates in early child development programs: "among the 14-year-olds, only 4% had attended preschool programs specifically designed for Aboriginal children when they were preschoolers. At the time of survey in 2001, 16% of six-year-old Aboriginal children in non-reserve areas had attended preschool programs specifically designed for them" (Statistics Canada, 2001c). As these statistics show, Aboriginal children's attendance at preschool is greatly distributed – both in terms of year they were born and Aboriginal ancestry. This is demonstrated for non-reserve communities in the figure below.

Figure 5. Aboriginal children in non-reserve areas who ever attended preschool programs, Canada, 2001

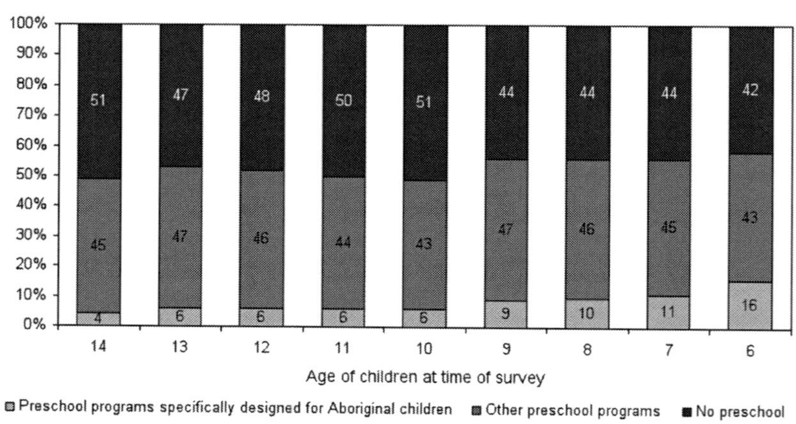

Source: (Statistics Canada, 2001c).

Note: Percentages in Figure 5 may not add up to 100% due to rounding.

Figure 5 on the previous page, which is posted on Statistics Canada's website (Statistics Canada, 2001c) shows that there has been a four-fold increase over eight years in the proportion of Aboriginal children in non-reserve areas attending preschool programs designed for them. Despite these gains, the absolute numbers remain low: "while one in two Aboriginal children in non-reserve areas attended preschool programs, only one in six attended programs specifically designed for them" (Statistics Canada, 2001c). Since there was no statistically significant change over the number of Aboriginal children attending general preschool programs (i.e. not Aboriginal-specific programs), there is reason to believe that the potential for growth and development in this area comes through tailored programming. The hope is that such programs will encourage greater participation in early childhood education and allow children to gain important social and intellectual skills – both of which are integral for ensuring their long-term well-being and functioning in the world. It is also believed that such programs will prepare children for school later in life and reduce drop out rates among Aboriginal high school students. In fact, researchers (Cairns, Cairns, & Neckerman, 1989) have shown that high school dropout rates are linked to a child's first five years at school. This further suggests that education and learning, especially in an individual's early years, may be a key to individual success and community prosperity (Cardinal, Schopflocher, Svenson, Morrison, & Laing, 2004).

5.4 Parental Smoking and Household Smoke

As has been discussed earlier in this book, environmental factors can influence one's risk for chronic diseases at all life stages. It is important to note, however, that certain groups are more vulnerable to household environments. Children are one such group: children both spend more time indoors and are exposed to the household during their development, which in turn influences the impact of environmental exposures. This is because long-term exposures to environmental risk factors can have harmful effects on growth, development, and function later in life (Sin, et al., 2004). For the purposes of this section, the impact of traditional and non-traditional tobacco use, as well as coal and wood-burning stoves will be discussed.

Tobacco use is often discussed in terms of individual habits and practices. As such, it is often forgotten that the habits and practices of parents and other caregivers can impact their child health and development after infancy. While the prevalence and impact of smoking on an individual is discussed in the adulthood and adolescent sections, the focus here is the impact of second-hand smoke on children. It is well documented that habitual smoking and passive smoking are significant problems in many Aboriginal communities. As a result, studies have found that many Aboriginal children live in homes where one or both of the parents smoke. This is particularly common for children with respiratory and other chronic ailments. For example, a study of First Nations children, 73% of those reporting airway obstruction lived in a home where one or both of the parents smoked (Orr, McDonald, Milley, & Brown, 2001). High parental smoking rates were also documented in a 1995-96 study of bronchiolitis among Inuit children: parental smoking occurred in 42 households (48.8%) of the 86 children studied and parents reported smoking within the vicinity of the house in another 31 households; parents in only three households claimed to be non-smokers (Mann, Wadsworth, & Colley, 1992). It is not surprising, therefore, that the literature also demonstrates that smoking exacerbates early life risks for chronic respiratory diseases (Millar, 1992; Sin, Wells, Svenson, & Man, 2002). The physiological reasoning behind this is that smoke causes damage to the respiratory system that encourages or progresses the development of chronic respiratory problems (Alwyn, 2004). As the effects of smoking accumulate over the life course, exposure to smoke at a young age causes great risk for the development of chronic diseases associated with smoking, such as diabetes, cardiovascular diseases, and respiratory conditions, later in life. As such, the living environment and conditions that children are exposed to, through their parents' lifestyle choices and their home environments are important to consider. The influence of household smoke is briefly discussed below.

The potential of household smoke other than direct parental smoking is enhanced by the continued use of coal and wood-burning stoves in many communities and the poor structural integrity of many Aboriginal homes, which can enable outdoor smoke to enter the home (Cardinal, et al., 2004; Petersen, Singleton, & Leonard, 2003). Like passive smoke, household smoke can greatly aggravate the pulmonary system and interrupt normal breathing patterns or the growth, development, and function of the lungs and other organs of the pulmonary system (Harris, Glazier, Eng, & McMurray, 1998). In short, the association between poor air quality, the use of wood-burning stoves, poor housing conditions, and poor child respiratory health in many Aboriginal communities cause reason for concern (Chronic Disease Prevention Alliance of Canada, 2006).

6. Childhood and Adolescent Risk Factors

While the early stages of development in childhood are important to consider with regard to one's health and well-being throughout life, so too is the health of an individual throughout childhood and adolescence. As early childhood represents an important stage of development and growth, so do the physical developments (sexual and body changes) that occur during adolescence. Furthermore, the important psychological and social changes that occur alongside the physical changes mark this period as a critical stage towards becoming an adult. Key risk factors, such as obesity, smoking and physical inactivity continue to be over-represented among Aboriginal children and youth compared to the Canadian national average (Guo, Roche, Chumlea, Gardner, & Siervogel, 1994; Serdula, et al., 1993). Thus, health risk profile of this cohort is integral to consider from a life course perspective.

6.1 Childhood Obesity

Longitudinal studies among non-Aboriginal people have shown that being overweight or obese during childhood and adolescence is linked with childhood diabetes and predicts adult obesity (Barrett-Connor, 1989), which is associated with type 2 diabetes (Hubert, Feinleib, McNamara, & Castelli, 1983) and coronary heart disease (Kumanyika, 1993). While high rates of pediatric obesity have been reported in studies of several racial groups (Bernard, Lavallee, Gray-Donald, & Delisle, 1995), Aboriginal children have been found to have a particularly high rates (Tjepkema, 2002): several studies have shown that Aboriginal children weigh (on average) more than other Canadians (T. K. Young, Dean, Flett, & Wood-Steiman, 2000). In a study of First Nations children aged 4 to 19, alarming obesity prevalence rates were documented: 64% of female children and 60% of male children were reported as being obese. In this study, obese children were shown to have an increased risk for diabetes. It is critical to note here, however, that in Aboriginal children living in the arctic, BMI should be interpreted with caution, because these children display a different pattern of growth with a high-weight-for-height pattern needed to survive in the climate they live in (MacMillan, et al., 1996). This different pattern of growth should not be confused with obesity (Reilly, et al., 2005).

In order to understand the etiology of Aboriginal childhood obesity, it is important to examine the root causes discussed in the Aboriginal and non-Aboriginal literature. An English longitudinal study conducted by Reilly et al. (2005) carefully examined early life risk factors for childhood obesity. In addition to the associations of childhood obesity with high birth weight and parental obesity, researchers found that children who watched television for more than 8 hours a week were at an increased risk of being obese (Reilly, et al., 2005). Sleep duration was also independently associated with childhood obesity: children in the lowest two quarters of sleep duration (<10.5 hours and 10.5-10.9 hours) at 30 months were more likely to be obese at age 7 than children in the highest quarter (>12 hours). The reasoning behind this correlation is that while television viewing reduces energy expenditure, sleep duration alters growth hormone secretion; changes a child's exposure to obesity-promoting factors, such as evening food intake, and acts as a marker for adequate physical activity levels (A. J. Hanley, et al., 2000).

A study undertaken in the Sandy Lake First Nations community also examined the correlation between obesity and television viewing. This study found that children who watched more than five hours of television per day were associated with a 2.5-fold increase in the risk of becoming (or being) overweight, when compared to children who watched less than 2 hours of television per day (A. J. Hanley, et al., 2000). In the same study, children with higher fitness levels and greater fiber intake were less likely to be overweight (First Nations Centre, 2004). According to the 1997 First Nations and Inuit Regional Health Survey, 98% of children watched television each week for an average of 2.9 hours each day (Bernard, et al., 1995; Ng, Marshall, & Willows, 2006). Other Aboriginal studies have reported that overweight Cree schoolchildren and adolescents participated in significantly less physical activity and consumed significantly fewer servings of fruits and vegetables than did their normal weight peers (First Nations Centre, 2004). When asked by the RHS about the availability of sports and cultural facilities in their community, fewer than half of Ontario Aboriginal youth reported having sports facilities. The most commonly cited needs were for a community swimming pool, followed by playground equipment, arena and drop-in centres (Ritchie & Reading, 2004). As issues of obesity in Aboriginal communities across the nation relate to an increasingly sedentary lifestyle, a lack of exercise, and poor nutrition, these underlying predictors of obesity should be better understood and targeted for prevention. Such intervention is important because it is likely that reductions in pediatric obesity will enable substantial positive health changes later in life.

6.2 Smoking

Even though smoking rates have declined among Aboriginal Peoples in recent years, Aboriginal smoking rates are still higher than those in the non-Aboriginal population (Chronic Disease Prevention Alliance of Canada, 2006; Ritchie & Reading, 2004). A significant concern, however, are the high rates of smoking among Aboriginal children and youth (Health Canada, 2003b).

Aboriginal youth are smoking at much higher rates than their Canadian counterparts. For Canadian youth, the prevalence of smoking, was found to be 18% for 15-19 year olds and 30% for young adults aged 20-24, with higher rates for female smokers (First Nations Centre). Comparatively, the prevalence of tobacco smoking among Aboriginal youth, reported by the 1991 Aboriginal Peoples Survey (2002/03), was 54% among 15–19 year olds and 65% among 20–24 year olds. Inuit youth were most likely to smoke (73% in the 15–24 age group) compared to the Métis or First Nations youth (56% and 59% respectively in the 15–24 age group). The distribution of smoking patterns among different age groups and genders is illustrated in Figure 6.

Figure 6. The Distribution of Smoking Patterns Among Different Ages (n=2,494)

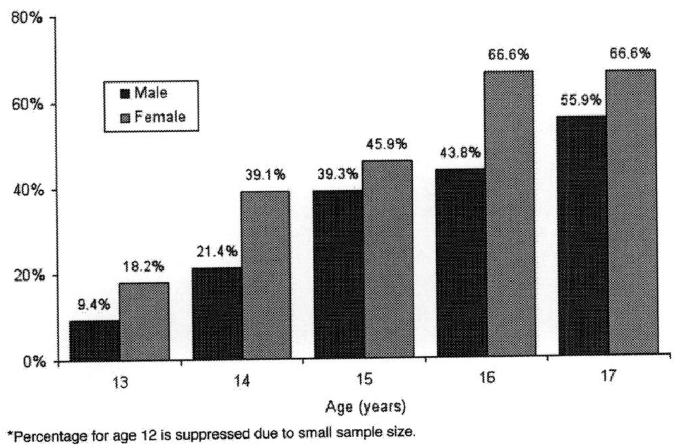

Source: (First Nations Centre, 2004).

High rates of smoking among Aboriginal teenagers are of particular concern for the future health of the Aboriginal population because they represent the largest demographic group within the Aboriginal population and because they represent the future of this population. Particularly high rates of smoking among females suggest the need to target this group and understand the particular causes associated with this gender difference.

In addition to high prevalence rates, Aboriginal smokers have been found to initiate smoking at an earlier age. According to reports by parents in Manitoba, 19% of all Aboriginal children under the age of 18 smoke and the peak age for starting smoking was 16 years, with many Aboriginal youth beginning as young as age 11. A survey conducted at the 2002 North American Indigenous Games found that Aboriginal youth (between the ages of 12-22) reported an average age of 12.2 years for smoking initiation, with the youngest reported age being 4 years old (Ritchie & Reading, 2004). By the age of 6, about 2% of Aboriginal youth smokers had initiated smoking, initiation rates continued to increase every year until peaking at age 12 when 20% of current youth smokers began smoking (Mann, et al., 1992). Overall, the research shows that Aboriginal children today start smoking at a very young age.

Beginning smoking at such a young age means that these children have virtually an entire lifetime to accumulate risks for chronic diseases associated with smoke-related environments and activities. It is well-documented that smoking exacerbates early life risks for respiratory diseases by damaging the respiratory system and encouraging or progressing the development of chronic respiratory problems (Cunningham, Dockery, Gold, & Speizer, 1995). Throughout childhood and later in life, exposure to smoke can continue to reduce lung function and increase the risk of respiratory problems (Retnakaran, Hanley, Connelly, Harris, & Zinman, 2005). The consistently high rates of smoking among Aboriginal youth also raise concerns about the long-term risks of developing chronic conditions. A study of the Sandy Lake First Nation, which reported that 82% of participants between the ages of 15 and 19 currently smoked (Ellickson, 2001), found a strong association between current smoking exposure and cardiovascular risk factors. This means that both immediate and long-term implications are an issue for this population.

Research shows, however, that smoking also affects one's mental health. A longitudinal, five-year follow-up study has found a statistically significant ($p<0.05$) association between early smoking and high-risk behaviours in grade-seven adolescents (Ellickson, 2001): compared with non-smokers, early smokers were 82 times more likely to engage in weekly marijuana use and 36 times more likely to engage in hard drug use; 11 times more likely to engage in weekly drinking and eight times more likely to engage in binge drinking; seven times more likely to steal. These adolescents were also at higher risk for low academic achievement and behavioural problems at school and engage in predatory and relational violence (First Nations Centre, 2005).

Despite the overwhelmingly negative statistics reported in the literature on Aboriginal youth smoking, there are also positive statistics regarding the smoking practices of this population. For example, the 2002/03 RHS reported that Aboriginal youth smoke significantly less cigarettes a day than Canadian youth in the fifth to nine grades age group (5.9 vs. 8.1 cigarettes a day) (First Nations Centre, 2005). A cross-sectional, opportunistic study conducted at the North American Indigenous Games (NAIG) in Winnipeg, Canada, found the prevalence of tobacco smoking in the studied cohort of 570 Aboriginal youth between ages 12 to 22 years old was 32% (Ritchie & Reading, 2004). A follow-up study conducted at the Cowichan 2008 NAIG, measured an even lower rate of smoking in Aboriginal youth: only 6.3% of youth were currently smokers (Kelly, Link, & Reading, 2009). This lower prevalence rate suggests that because the participants were attending or competing at a sports event they may be more health conscious than other Aboriginal youth and, therefore, may be less likely to develop unhealthy lifestyle behaviours (B. C. Canada, 2001). As such, more participation in sport or other health activities may be an effective way to improve smoking rates in Aboriginal communities. Finally, a 3 % reduction in smoking rates among First Nations adults living in Canada from 1997-2001 (First Nations and Inuit Regional Health Survey National Steering Committee, 1999; First Nations Centre, 2005) is encouraging for the future. The hope is that declines in smoking rates among adults with continue and will also influence lower smoking rates among children and youth through positive role modelling. At the very least, however, Aboriginal children and youth will likely be exposed to less passive smoke.

Issues related to passive smoking are important to consider for this age group, just as they are for infants and throughout early childhood (see natal and early childhood sections for "parental smoking"). According to the Tobacco Use in British Columbia 1997 survey, 32% of Aboriginal children were daily or nearly daily exposed to cigarette smoking in their homes. This compares to 18 % of all BC households with children exposed to smoking (B. C. Canada, 2001). The data from this survey is summarized in Figure 7 below.

Figure 7. Exposure to Second-Hand Smoke Households with Children Age 11 and Under, BC, 199

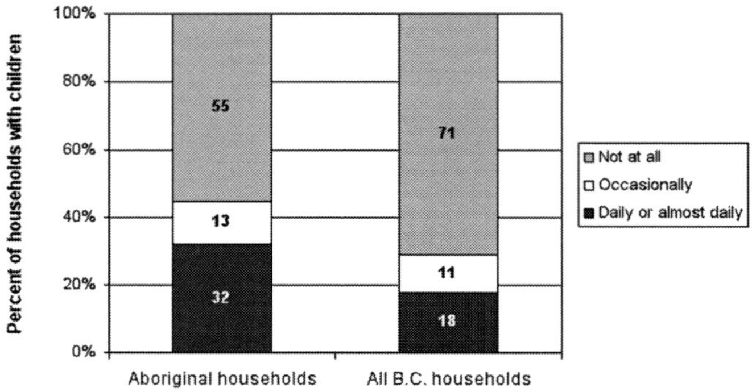

Source: (Orr, et al., 2001).

As noted earlier, extremely high parental smoking rates have been documented in studies of Inuit children: parental smoking occurred in 48.8% of the homes and parents reported smoking within the vicinity of 36% of the households; parents in only 3.4% of the households claimed to be non-smokers (Koch, et al., 2003). Although the correlation between passive smoking and chronic disease development is not as clear as personal smoking behaviours, it has been found that passive smoking can complicate respiratory and other health problems and foster the development of chronic conditions. The varied influence of exposure to tobacco smoke on chronic disease is demonstrated by a study of 2273 American adolescents (Weitzman, et al., 2005). This study specifically examined the connection between smoking and metabolic syndrome. Out of the study population, 5.6% of the adolescents met the criteria for metabolic syndrome. However, the prevalence for metabolic syndrome, a clustering of risks for diabetes and cardio vascular disease. was 1.2% for those not exposed to tobacco smoke, 5.4% for those exposed to environmental tobacco smoke, and 8.7% for active smokers (First Nations Centre, 2005).

6.3 Sexual Health

According to RHS 2002-03, First Nations youth are more sexually active than their Canadian counterparts (First Nations Centre, 2005). Considering that "the levels of alcohol and drug abuse among First Nations youth are

[also] higher than those in mainstream society", it can be posited that First Nations youth could be at an increased risk of unprotected sexual activity and, therefore, sexually transmitted infections (Gray, 2005). The sexual health of Aboriginal youth is also related to the trends of cancer development. This is because it has been documented that women who have multiple sexual partners or who become sexually active at an early age are more likely to develop cervical cancer. The reason early sexual activity is linked to cancer risk is because during puberty cervical tissue undergoes many changes that might make the area more vulnerable to damage. There is also a suspected connection between sexually transmitted diseases (STD) and cervical cancer: "[i]nfection with human papilloma virus (HPV) increases your risk 20 to 100 times" (Gray, 2005). While HPV is a quite common sexually transmitted infection, there are over 100 types of HPV and only a few that are the high-risk types that will influence the risk of cervical cancer (Gray, 2005; NAHO, 2004; PapScreen Victoria, 2006). Nonetheless, sexual activity increases the risk of getting HPV and, in particular, high-risk types of HPV and, therefore, must be treated with caution and concern. While Pap smears have been shown to dramatically reduce the number of women who die from cervical cancer, traditionally low rates of Pap smear testing among Aboriginal women remains a concern for early detection and cancer survival in this population (Ontario Federation of Indian Friendship Centres, 2004).

Because of particular vulnerabilities among Aboriginal youth, such as low socioeconomic status, disempowerment as a result of historical and cultural conditions and lack of education, sexual exploitation is also a concern for this population's sexual health and well-being. Save the Children Canada's National Aboriginal Project released a report on the nature and depth of commercial sexual exploitation of Aboriginal children and youth across Canada. The study found that:

(1) the rate of commercial exploitation of Aboriginal children and youth has reached levels of more than 90% in some communities where the Aboriginal population is less than 10%; (2) the serious over-representation of Aboriginal youth in the sex trade is directly linked to the unacceptably high level of risk factors which Aboriginal children and youth face, including alarmingly high poverty rates (Ontario Federation of Indian Friendship Centres, 2004).

As described by the report, the reality of the disproportionately high rate of Aboriginal children and youth living in the sex trade is perpetuated by pressures related to poverty and low socioeconomic status common within this group (Chansonneuve, 2005). In addition to economic reasons, cultural and historical factors are essential to understanding the experiences of children and youth. In particular, the experiences of parents that are inherited by their children have been shown to have a lasting impact on the sexual health practices of Aboriginal children and youth. The particular impacts of the historic and current education system on the learned and experienced history of Aboriginal children and youth are discussed in greater detail below.

6.4 Education

The education system, past and present, is an integral aspect of the lives of Aboriginal youth and adolescents. Looking to the past first, this section will discuss the legacy of the residential school and its ongoing impacts on health. Next, the experiences of Aboriginal peoples in the current school system and their impacts on health will be discussed.

6.4.1 Residential Schools

Education of Indians (now known as First Nations) became a responsibility of the federal government in 1867 under the British North America Act (Chansonneuve, 2005; Fournier & Crey, 1997). By this time, Indian day schools had been established, but the government was urged by the Davin report of 1879 to establish residential schools instead: Davin believed residential schools to be the most effective means of assimilating Indian children. In 1892, the Canadian government established partnerships with Roman Catholic, Anglican, Presbyterian and Methodist churches to run the operation of Indian residential schools. Except in the provinces of Newfoundland, Prince Edward Island, and New Brunswick, residential schools were established across the country (Fournier & Crey, 1997). Attendance increased after 1920, when an amendment to the Indian Act made education of Indian children between the ages of 7 and 15 years old mandatory for ten months of the year (Fournier & Crey, 1997). Nearly three-quarters of Indian children across Canada were attending residential school by 1930. Some Aboriginal children began attending provincially-run public day schools in the 1950s, and by 1969, when the federal government took full control over residential schools, 60% of Aboriginal students attended public day schools (Fournier & Crey, 1997). From the inception of residential schools in the 1800s to the closure of most of the schools in the 1970s, almost one-third of Aboriginal children spent a large portion of their childhood in attendance at residential school (Beauchamp, et al., 2004; Chansonneuve, 2005). The last federally run residential school closed in 1996 (Dion Stout & Harp, 2007). There are an estimated 86,000 residential school survivors alive today (Dion Stout & Harp, 2007; King, 2006).

The residential school system was not exclusive to Indian children. The boarding, missionary, hostel and residential schools attended by Inuit children are also defined as part of the residential school system;[5] further, Inuit children who lived away from home while attending federal day schools are considered residential school survivors. In some areas of the North, churches ran federally funded missionary schools until the federal government accepted responsibility of Inuit education (King, 2006). Education in the Arctic was controlled by the federal government between 1955 and 1970. Inuit student enrolment rose from a total of 549 in 1956 to 2,390 in 1963 (Chansonneuve, 2005). Less than 15% of Inuit children aged 6 to 15 years were enrolled in school in 1955, but by 1964, three-quarters (75%) were enrolled.

Métis children were also students of the residential school system. Exact enrolment numbers are difficult to determine because records of Métis students were not always kept (Chartrand, 2006). Although Métis education was not recognized as a federal responsibility, Métis children were occasionally allowed to enroll or enrolled in residential schools for a particular purpose (Chansonneuve, 2005; Chartrand, 2006; Logan, 2001), such as assimilation or to boost attendance records in order to receive more funding (Chansonneuve, 2005; Logan, 2001). Factors that influenced the likelihood of Métis admission to residential schools included proximity of schools to Métis communities, school denomination (as Métis had a stronger connection to the Roman Catholic Church), family history, and social standing (Logan, 2001). Métis children were more often admitted to residential school if their family had money to pay for schooling, if their physical features were characteristic of Indian attributes, or if their lifestyle was most associated with that of Indians and, therefore, seen to be in greater need of assimilation (Fournier & Crey, 1997; Kirmayer, Simpson, & Cargo, 2003; Reading, 1999).

5 The residential school system in Canada has been defined to include "industrial schools, boarding school, homes for students, hostels, billets, residential schools, and residential schools with a majority of day students or a combination of any of the above".

Punishments and abuse were widespread and often severe in the residential school system. Children who expressed Aboriginal language and culture or sought contact with family were commonly administered harsh disciplines, which some scholars have even labelled as torture (Chrisjohn & Young, 1995). Such punishments exceeded the standard forms of discipline in Canadian public schools at the time and "the infractions which 'warranted' this treatment were not infractions for any children in Canada save Aboriginal ones" (Chansonneuve, 2005). The abuse that occurred at residential schools included physical, sexual, emotional and spiritual abuse and has been described as ritualized, or "repeated, systematic, sadistic and humiliating trauma" (Chansonneuve, 2005; Chrisjohn & Young, 1995; Fournier & Crey, 1997; Kirmayer, Simpson, & Cargo, 2003; Reading, 1999). Children were: under constant surveillance, continually underfed and malnourished, humiliated in front of peers, degraded for their Aboriginal culture and heritage, deprived of gifts and letters from family, denied emotional comfort, forced to perform hard labour, and forced to witness the abuse of other children (Fournier & Crey, 1997). Fournier and Crey (1997) stated that student deaths due to abuse and neglect were concealed, but had the schools been held accountable, they would be guilty of "criminal negligence, manslaughter and even murder" (Beauchamp, et al., 2004). In the 1990s, apologies were issued from the Catholic, Anglican, United and Presbyterian churches as well as the Canadian government for the physical and sexual abuses that occurred in residential schools (Corrado, Cohen, Aboriginal Healing Foundation (Canada), & Corrado Research and Evaluation Associates., 2003; Waldram, Herring, & Young, 2006). In June 2008, an apology was finally issued by the Canadian Government (Harper, 2008).

In addition to the multitude of abuses experienced in residential schools, children endured atrocious living conditions. Low government funding contributed to the poor nutritional value of food and lack of medical services available to students (Fournier & Crey, 1997). Dormitories of the schools were often overcrowded and unventilated (Corrado, et al., 2003; Fournier & Crey, 1997; Waldram, et al., 2006). As a result of the poor living conditions, illness and diseases such as tuberculosis raged through residential schools (Chrisjohn & Young, 1995; Fournier & Crey, 1997).

The goal of the residential school system to assimilate, rather than educate, Indian children is demonstrated by the poor quality of education provided.

Only half of the day at school was devoted to academic instruction, while the rest of the day was spent in teaching children religious ideology or forcing children to contribute to school maintenance and other labour-intensive projects (Fournier & Crey, 1997). In 1930, at the height of residential school operations, three-quarters (75%) of Indian students were below third grade level (compared to less than half of the children in provincial public schools), and only 3% of Indian students achieved higher than a sixth grade education (compared to one-third of children in provincial public schools) (Reading, 1999). The inadequate education provided by residential schools left former students with few skills to function in mainstream society and may have adversely affected their future quality of life (Chartrand, 2006; King, 2006; Logan, 2001).

Experiences of Métis and Inuit children who attended residential schools were often similar to those of Indian children. Stories of neglect, poor living conditions, fierce punishments, cultural suppression and physical and sexual abuse have been told by Métis and Inuit residential school survivors (Logan, 2001). Some Métis students adjusted more easily to residential school life because of their greater familiarity with Catholicism and the English or French languages (Chartrand, 2006; Logan, 2001). Other Métis children felt they were treated as "second class" students because the federal government did not provide funding to churches for education of the Métis and they were considered neither full-blooded Indians with recognized rights, nor full-blooded Caucasians of dominant society (J. Anderson, 2003).

The residential school system is a dark chapter in the history of Canada's treatment of Aboriginal peoples and their educational history. What it does so effectively highlight, however, is the great impact that educational settings can have on children, parents, grandparents, and, indeed, generations. As we look to the current educational system, it will be important to remember the history of the residential school system, as well as the close connection that education has on the economic and social success of all Canadians.

6.4.2 The Current Education System

In general, data shows that school attendance of Aboriginal youth is lower than non-Aboriginal youth. For instance, data from 1996 shows that "68% of Aboriginal youth were in school compared to 83% of non-Aboriginal youth". School completion has also been shown to be lower: in 1996, just over half (52%) of the Aboriginal population aged 20 to 24 living in non-reserve areas had not completed secondary school. By 2001, this proportion had dropped to 48% compared to 26% of the non-Aboriginal population (Statistics Canada, 2001c).

The proportion of secondary school graduates is an important predictor of future education and employment rates. Some important information on Aboriginal post-secondary enrolment and completion rates is included in a report completed by the Millennium Scholarship Foundation in 2004, titled "Aboriginal Peoples and Post-Secondary Education: What Educators have learned." Some of its key points are reviewed in the following paragraph.

As noted by the Millennium Scholarship Foundation, post-secondary enrolment and completion rates for Aboriginal peoples have been steadily increasing over the past two decades. Despite these increases, however, the rates for Aboriginal peoples remain significantly lower than those of non-Aboriginal Canadians (Malatest, 2004). For instance, the 1996 Census found that registered Indians and other Aboriginal peoples were less likely than all other Canadians to have obtained a university degree (3% and 4% versus 14% respectively) as well as being less likely to have some post-secondary education (37% and 47% versus 51% respectively) (Malatest, 2004).

While the increasing numbers of Aboriginal graduates is encouraging, it is important to remember that there are still many limitations and barriers to Aboriginal youth's educational achievements. Thus, post-secondary education must take into account the social, cultural or economic needs of Aboriginal peoples (Malatest, 2004). The following quote outlines some of these limitations and barriers:

> While socio-economic factors such as poverty and unemployment put them at an obvious disadvantage, Aboriginal students also face more subtle barriers such as discrimination, low self-concept and institutional insensitivity to Aboriginal cultures. Many Aboriginal students arrive in post-secondary institutions without adequate high school preparation; others struggle to balance education with family responsibilities. Combined with a history of forced assimilation through educational institutions, the barriers to Aboriginal participation in post-secondary education are formidable (Malatest, 2004).

These challenges and barriers, as well as the raw numbers on Aboriginal education, are important to take into account, as the importance and value of a formal secondary and post-secondary education is only increasing with time: "With the advent of the knowledge-based economy, jobs are becoming increasingly scarce for individuals without a diploma or a degree from a high school, college or university" (Statistics Canada, 2001c). Statistics Canada (2001c) found that differences in unemployment rates among Aboriginal Peoples could be partially attributed to educational backgrounds. This means that education can predict the employability of a person and, therefore, also their future socioeconomic status.

Research has also found that education rates among Aboriginal children and youth is closely related to their parents' education levels (Statistics Canada, 2001c). For instance, De Broucker and Lavallée (1998) have reported that the higher parental education levels, the higher the education levels of their children. This association is demonstrated in the figure below, which shows that parental education is a factor in Aboriginal children's likelihood of repeating a grade.

Figure 8. Percentage of non-reserve Aboriginal children repeating a grade

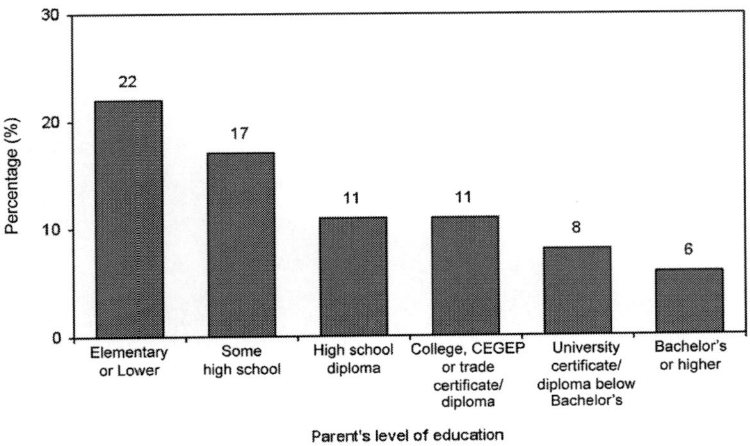

Source: (Statistics Canada, 2001c).

The figure shows that as the parent's education level increases, the proportion of children having ever repeated a grade decreases. That is, for parents who had not gone beyond elementary school, one out of five of their children had repeated a grade, whereas only 6% of children of parents with a bachelor's degree or higher had repeated a grade at some point in their life.

Some reasons given for the correlation between child and parent education include: (1) parents with higher levels of educational attainment will take greater interest in their child's education and, therefore, encourage learning activities and homework (Stevenson & Baker, 1987) and (2) highly educated patents tend to have higher academic expectations for their children, which has shown to greatly influence the success of a child in school (Astone & McClanahan, 1991; Hull, Research, Analysis, & Indian and Northern Affairs, 2000; Teachman, 1987; Teachman & Paasch, 1998). In addition to parental influences, the extended family, Elders and the community play key roles in childhood education and learning in Aboriginal populations. This is because learning in Aboriginal communities includes both cognitive development and learning how to behave in society (G. D. Smith, Hart, Blane, Gillis, & Hawthorne, 1997). This suggests that the educational levels and supports provided by the community and the extended family are all important for childhood growth and development.

In addition to parental and family educational levels and support, the success of children in school has also been linked to their family's household income. That is, many studies have shown that children from economically disadvantaged families experience greater difficulties learning and have more problems in school (Chao & Willms, 2002; Duncan & Brooks-Gunn, 1997; Petterson & Albers, 2001; Ross & Roberts, 2000; J. R. Smith & Klebanov, 1997; Statistics Canada, 2001c). Statistics showing education levels in Aboriginal children living in non-reserve areas verifies this understanding: "About 16% of children in families with income below the low income cut-off had repeated a school year at some point, compared with only 10% of children in families at or above the low income cut-off" (Bennett, Blackstock, & De La Ronde, 2005; Canada, 2006; Fournier & Crey, 1997; Gough, Trochmé, Brown, Knoke, & Blackstock, 2005; Kirmayer, et al., 2003; Sinclair, 2007).

6.5 Foster Care and State Wardship

In the 1960s, when an increasing number of Aboriginal children were being enrolled in provincial public schools rather than federally funded residential schools, a new assault on Aboriginal families emerged. Termed as the Sixties Scoop, this assault was propagated through a disproportionately high number of Aboriginal children being taken from their families and communities to be placed in out-of-home care (Fournier & Crey, 1997). Aboriginal children, who made up less than 4% of the Canadian population and who represented only 1% of children in care in 1959, suddenly represented 30-40% of children in care at the end of the 1960s (Fournier & Crey, 1997; Sinclair, 2007). More often than not, Aboriginal children taken from their families were placed in non-Aboriginal homes (Fournier & Crey, 1997; Gough, et al., 2005; Royal Commission on Aboriginal Peoples, 1996) reported that except in Quebec, the proportion of Aboriginal children in care placed in non-Aboriginal homes was 70 to 90% across provinces. Much like children who attended residential schools, Aboriginal children who became legal wards were separated from their parents, siblings, communities and cultural identity, often without the knowledge of where they came from and sometimes without their birth names (Bennett, Blackstock, & De La Ronde, 2005). Siblings were often placed in separate homes, partially due to the difficulty of finding homes to accommodate large Aboriginal families, but also with the goal of better assimilating the children. Few children were ever returned to their home (Fournier & Crey, 1997).

Driven by the same paternalistic attitude that created the residential school system, the Sixties Scoop was propelled forward with the belief that Aboriginal parents were unfit to raise their children (Canada, 2006a). The poor parenting skills that stemmed from generations of Aboriginal children attending residential schools likely contributed to this belief (Bennett, et al., 2005; Fournier & Crey, 1997). However, many children were taken from their homes for reasons Aboriginal parents had little control over; that is, poor socioeconomic status and simply being Aboriginal (K. Morris, 2007). Social workers, who were trained to uphold Eurocentric standards in child welfare, believed it in the best interest of the children to remove them from reserves stricken with poverty rather than provide support services to families and communities in need (Fournier & Crey, 1997; Kirmayer, Simpson, & Cargo, 2003).

Although this process of removing Aboriginal children from their homes has been termed the Sixties Scoop, child welfare agencies have continued to remove Aboriginal children from their homes long after the 1960s (Fournier & Crey, 1997). By the end of the 1970s, at least one in three Aboriginal children had been involved in government care (Bennett, et al., 2005). In 1983, Aboriginal children represented roughly 50% of children in care in Alberta, 60% in Manitoba, and 70% in Saskatchewan (Blackstock, Trochmé, & Bennett, 2004; Kirmayer, et al., 2003). Today, Aboriginal children are still disproportionately represented among children in out-of-home care (Sinclair, 2007), and one university professor has suggested that the Sixties Scoop has evolved into the "Millennium Scoop" (Blackstock, et al., 2004). Blackstock and colleagues (2004) estimate that when compared to the number of Aboriginal children in residential schools during years of peak enrolment, there are three times as many Aboriginal children in out-of-home care today. Fournier and Crey (1997) reported that in British Columbia, over half (52%) of children placed in care by court order each year are Aboriginal. Over three-quarters (78%) of Aboriginal children in permanent care in British Columbia are cared for in non-Aboriginal homes (Sinclair, 2007).

The outcomes for Aboriginal children raised in non-Aboriginal homes are not always negative, as some of those children have grown to find success and happiness in their careers, families and communities (Bennett, et al., 2005; Carriere, 2007; Sinclair, 2007). However, many Aboriginal survivors of the child welfare system have shared stories of their struggle to establish a sense of identity among foster and adoptive families, birth families, Aboriginal communities and mainstream society (Bennett, et al., 2005; Morris, 2007; Sinclair, 2007). These struggles have presented difficulties throughout their childhood and adolescence and sometimes into adulthood. The negative impacts on the mental health of Aboriginal children cared for in non-Aboriginal homes may include issues of identity formation, low self-esteem, feelings of shame, suicidal ideations and attempts, substance abuse, homelessness, and incarceration (J. Anderson, 2003). Not only have these mental health issues emerged as problems for the cohort of grown Aboriginal 'Sixties Scoop' survivors, but for the disproportionate number of Aboriginal children still a part of the child welfare system, they represent the potential for health problems of the near future.

7. Adulthood and the Elderly Risk Factors

As discussed in the previous sections, the Aboriginal population is younger than the non-Aboriginal population: "The median age among the Aboriginal population was 24.7 years in 2001, compared to 37.7 years for Canada's non-Aboriginal population" (Health Canada, 2003c). But, while adulthood does not command the population as much as the baby boomers do in Canada's non-Aboriginal population, their health needs and concerns are of equal importance. Further, as the life expectancy of Aboriginal peoples continues to increase and as chronic health conditions begin to take precedence over communicable diseases, the health and well being of adults and elders will begin to take an even more important role in the profile of Aboriginal health. With this in mind, the particular risk factors associated with chronic diseases among Aboriginal adults, such as smoking, alcohol abuse, obesity, and employment and education, are discussed further. Finally, the unique aspects of elder health are discussed at the end of this section.

7.1 Smoking

As noted in the sections on maternal smoking, parental smoking, and smoking among Aboriginal children and youth, the Aboriginal population has higher rates of smoking than the non-Aboriginal population. In fact, the Aboriginal population has a much higher proportion of current cigarette smokers (58% vs. 31%), and fewer former smokers (17% vs. 23%) or never smokers (24% vs. 45%) than the non-Aboriginal population. According to Health Canada's 2005 Tobacco Report, almost 60% of on-reserve First Nations adults aged 18-34 years smoke. The 2002/03 RHS documented similar smoking rates (58.8%) among First Nations adults (First Nations Centre, 2005). This can be compared with data from the Canadian Tobacco Use Monitoring Survey (CTUMS) which reported 21% of Canadian general population were smokers in 2003. The smoking rates are even higher among Inuit in the North of Canada, where about 66% of adult population smoke tobacco (Statistics Canada, 2008b).

What is important to add to these statistics is a discussion of the risks of chronic disease development associated with smoking. For instance, it has been estimated that smoking tobacco is responsible for about one third of all fatal cancers (Greenhalgh, 1981; Haustein, 2003; Swales & De Bono, 1993). The relationship between smoking rates and cancer rates has been established by the research community and found to be proportionally related: in other words, the higher the smoking rate, the higher the rate of cancer. This is of concern for Aboriginal cancer rates, as statistics have already begun to show rising rates of previously non-existent cancers in Aboriginal populations. Smoking has also been linked to an increased risk of cardiovascular disease and diabetes (Sin, Wells, Svenson, & Man, 2002), and a higher incidence and prevalence rates of chronic obstructive pulmonary disease and asthma (Ghadirian, 2005)

The good news is that changes to smoking habits at any life stage can greatly reduce the risks associated with smoking. As Ghadirian (2005) explains, quitting smoking can greatly reduce the risks of cardiovascular disease: within a year of quitting, a former smoker's risk of heart disease is reduced by nearly 50%, compared to someone who continues to smoke. A study conducted in men younger than age 55 revealed that while those who had quit smoking within the past year had a risk level not significantly different from current smokers, the risk declined after 2 years to nearly that of non-smokers (Ghadirian, 2005). The residual risk for cardiovascular disease following cessation is strongly dependent on total previous exposure to cigarette smoke, length of time without cigarettes, and the health status of the individual at the time of stopping. However, after 10 to 15 years without cigarettes, the health status of most former smokers is not significantly different from that of a lifelong non-smoker (Stephens & Health Canada, 1994). This means that targeted smoking cessation strategies have the potential to improve disease risk rates and encourage better health in the future (Tjepkema, 2002).

7.2 Alcohol Abuse

According to the 2002/2003 RHS, First Nations people are more likely to completely abstain from alcohol consumption than the non-First Nations population (34.4% vs. 20.7% respectively) as well as reporting a lower frequency of alcohol consumption; 17.8% reported drinking more than once per week versus 44% of the non-First Nations population. However, First Nations adults are more likely to be considered heavy drinkers (First Nations Centre, 2005). According to National Cancer Institute, heavy alcohol use is defined as consumption of five or more drinks on a single occasion (National Cancer Institute, 2002). The prevalence of heavy drinking on a weekly basis has been found to be higher in First Nations adults (16%) than in the general Canadian population (6.2%). Consequently, the risks of heavy drinking on health are a serious concern for Canada's Aboriginal population.

Heavy drinking has been reported to increase the risks of developing cancers. In particular, high levels of consumption have been found to markedly increase the risk of liver and colorectal cancers. Consumption of just one drink per day for women, or two drinks per day for men, has been associated with an increased risk of developing cancers of the mouth, larynx, pharynx, esophagus, and liver. Furthermore, women who have two drinks per day are at 25% higher risk of developing breast cancer than women who don't drink alcohol (National Cancer Institute, 2002). Finally, the combination of alcohol consumption and smoking greatly increases the risk of lung cancer.

As will be discussed in further detail (Part III, Section 7.2.4), alcohol abuse can be a chronic condition. Its association, often, with depression, historical experiences, trauma, and other unpleasant memories or current situations, demonstrates that alcoholism has a profound effect on one's health and ability to function in the world around them. Thus, not only can alcohol influence and place people at risk for chronic conditions, but also its potential status as a chronic condition can create ongoing difficulties and additional problems for the user. Physical and psychosocial risks associated with alcoholism, therefore, need to be taken very seriously both in Aboriginal and non-Aboriginal communities.

7.3 Obesity and Inactivity

Obesity is an important risk factor for many chronic diseases. Obesity is often measured through body weight measures and/or the body mass index (BMI), which produces a measure based on one's height and weight. The percent of individuals with normal, higher or lower body mass index in Aboriginal and Canadian populations, reported in the 2002/03 RHS, is summarized in the table below.

Table 3. Distribution body weight groups among adults, living in Canada

Body Mass Index	First Nations Adults	Canadian Adults
Normal	25.9%	49%
Overweight	37.0%	33%
Obese	31.2%	15%

Source: (First Nations Centre, 2005).

As also described in the 2002/03 RHS report, the distribution of obesity within the Aboriginal population is influenced by gender (First Nations Centre, 2005). For instance, men were found to be overrepresented in the group of overweight individuals, while Aboriginal women were more likely to be obese or morbidly obese individuals (MacMillan, et al., 1996). It is important to note here that there have been concerns with the measurement of obesity for some Aboriginal groups, such as the Inuit. As has been shown among young arctic children, different patterns of growth and different height-to-weight gradients, which remain throughout adulthood, can cause an individual to be measured as obese when they are not (First Nations and Inuit Regional Health Survey National Steering Committee, 1999). The 1999 First Nations and Inuit Regional Health Survey (First Nations and Inuit Regional Health Survey National Steering Committee, 1999) found that 36% of Labrador Inuit women and 26% of Labrador Inuit men are overweight (McIntyre & Shah, 1986). The prevalence of obesity in Aboriginal population of Northern Ontario ranges from 50% to 70% in Aboriginal women and 30% to 50% among Aboriginal men (T. K. Young & Sevenhuysen, 1989). A study within an Ojibwa-Cree population found that in some age and sex groups, almost 90% of those studied were overweight and obese (Tjepkema, 2002). Further, there appears to be very little difference between the physical activity levels of the off-reserve Aboriginal population and the non-Aboriginal population in Canada located in the provinces. In the territories, however, Aboriginal people were less likely to be active than other Northerners (Denny, 2005).

A key contributing factor to obesity in Aboriginal and non-Aboriginal populations is inactivity. Unfortunately rates of inactivity have been shown to be high in many Aboriginal communities. A study conducted in the United States in 2001 and 2002, which surveyed American Inuit and American Native (AI/AN) people's chronic disease risk factors, found that 37.2% of AI/AN reported no physical activity during their leisure time. The survey also found that 29.3% of the people surveyed were obese (OR=1.41) (First Nations Centre, 2005). Such inactivity has also been reported among the First Nations population. Reasons for reduced physical activity include; the loss of First Nations traditional lands and practices, such as hunting, trapping and fishing, a higher proportion of Aboriginal people have begun to lead more sedentary lifestyle, an adoption of a non-traditional (or so-called "Western[6]") diet by First Nations people after colonization. As a result of these and other socio-economic changes, such as extreme poverty, the percentage of inactive and obese individuals in First Nations communities

6 A Westernized diet is typically high in fat and protein and low in fiber.

has increased (Statistics Canada, 2001a). The proportion of inactive and obese individuals is growing, however obesity can be prevented by education about the importance of exercise and the promotion of active living. Research needs to focus on healthy intervention strategies at the community.

7.4 Employment and Education

Because the average age of the Aboriginal population is 10 years younger than the non-Aboriginal population, significant increases are expected in the absolute number and relative proportion of Aboriginal working-age population (25-44 years) over the next decade. The level of education for this age group has improved by 14 per cent over the last decade, greater than the 10% seen among the non-Aboriginal population. However the gap between the two groups remains great (Malatest, 2004). For example, the proportion of Aboriginal people in their twenties with a post-secondary degree or diploma rose from 19% to 23% between 1981 and 1996, but the proportion of those with a university degree or certificate did not increase significantly (3% to 4%). Further still, education levels for Aboriginal peoples remain below the national average: in 1996, 54% of the Aboriginal population aged 15 and over did not have a high-school diploma, compared to 35% of the non-Aboriginal population (J. Anderson, 2003); in 2001, only 8% of Aboriginal peoples between the ages of 25-34 years had completed a university degree, compared to 28% of all other Canadians (Australia. Department of Employment Education and Training, 1990). Education levels and employment rates are closely associated with one another (Tjepkema, 2002). As a whole, Aboriginal peoples living off-reserve have lower levels of academic completion, household income and year-round employment than non-Aboriginal people (Statistics Canada, 2001c).

According to the 2001 Census, the unemployment rate for Aboriginal adults aged 25 to 34 with university degrees was 8%, while that for those who had completed grade 9 but not high school was 28%. For those who had not completed grade 9 the unemployment rate was 40% (Statistics Canada, 2001c). Researchers have also found that post-secondary educational attainment has some major positive influences on employment and earnings for Aboriginal peoples (Hull, Research, Analysis, & Indian and Northern Affairs, 2000; Maxim, White, Whitehead, & Beavon, 2000).

Statistics on Aboriginal unemployment highlight the magnitude of this significant problem: in 1998, the average unemployment rate on Aboriginal reserves was 29%, which is also almost triple the national rate (Canada. Parliament. House of Commons. Standing Committee on Health, 1995; Statistics Canada, 2001a). The situation was even worse in some communities, where unemployment rates were reported to be as high as 90% (MacMillan, et al., 1996). While some of the highest rates of unemployment can be found on-reserve, an average of 25% of Aboriginal adults (ages 15+) in 1996 were thought to be unemployed, as compared with just under 10% of the mainstream population (Statistics Canada, 2001a). The disparity in employment and its links to poverty is exemplified by the fact that in 1995, the average employment income of Aboriginal peoples was $17,382, which is about 1.5 times lower than the national average of $26,474 (MacMillan, et al., 1996). In 1990, more than half (54%) of adult Aboriginal people reported annual incomes below $10,000, while only 35 % of Canadians reported the same level of income (First Nations Centre, 2005; Oberle & INAC, 1993). More recent data has shown some improvements in employment rates of First Nations living in Canada: the 2002/03 RHS showed that 33.2% of First Nations adults reported their income below $10,000 and the overall employment rate of First Nations people was registered at 8 % lower that that of Canadian population in 2001 (First Nations Centre, 2005; Mendelson, 2004). More recent data have shown 5 to 7% improvement in employment rates from 1991 to 2000, and an equalization of employment rates among Aboriginal people living on- and off-reserve (Green, Blanchard, Young, & Griffith, 2003).

While these statistics paint an interesting picture of the socioeconomic landscape of Aboriginal peoples in Canada, it is important to highlight here that while education and employment directly impact one's socioeconomic status, they also have a particular impact on one's health and well-being. In fact, it has been found that education and employment can be key predictors of chronic disease development and survival. For example, lower cancer survival rates have been linked to low income levels and high unemployment rates (Ward, et al., 2004). A 2003 study found substantial clustering of diabetes in areas of Winnipeg with low socioeconomic status, poor environmental quality, poor lifestyles and high concentration Aboriginal peoples (Green, Blanchard, et al., 2003). The study also found that education and income were stronger predictors of diabetes than Aboriginal status, suggesting that socioeconomic status, rather than genetic factors were responsible for the high prevalence of diabetes (Health Canada, 2005a).

7.5 Elder Health

In Canada, life expectancy at birth for the "registered Indian" population and Inuit-inhabited regions remains significantly lower than that of the overall Canadian population (see Table 4).

Table 4. Life expectancy (in years) for Canada (200-2002), Registered Indians (2001) and Inuit-inhabited regions (1999-2003) as a function of gender

	Canada	Registered Indians	Inuit-inhabited Regions
Males	77.0	70.4 (gap – 6.6 years)	64.4 (gap – 12.6 years)
Females	82.0	75.5 (gap – 6.5 years)	69.8 (gap – 12.2 years)

Source: (Health Canada, 2009).

Elders comprise a smaller population of elderly people, and are generally younger in Aboriginal communities than non-Aboriginal communities. A distinction must be made between those who are elderly by age and those who are considered "Elders" in their communities because of the strength and wisdom that they hold. While age may run parallel to the classification of being an Elder, the experience, knowledge, and wisdom that the person has is far superior. In this section the health of the elderly and elders in Aboriginal populations will be discussed briefly in terms of being defined as the older subset of the population.

Not surprisingly, the risks attributed to elders' health are largely a result of increased age. Yet, because of a generally lower life expectancy and younger population, the particularities of the health of the older Aboriginal population and the risks associated with later life and chronic diseases has not been robustly explored in the literature. What has been noted in the Canadian literature is that one in three older Native Americans lived below the poverty level (Cueller, 1990). This means that many elderly Aboriginal people continue to struggle with low socioeconomic status and, therefore, likely do not have the financial resources to help manage and control the inevitable challenges in health conditions that come with age. This raises concern not only for the health and well-being of the elderly in Aboriginal populations, but also their basic subsistence and ability to survive without supplementary monetary support. It also raises concerns for the community: because Elders traditionally play such an important role in Aboriginal communities, the loss of their strength and ability to engage in cultural activities because of monetary or health conditions are concerning. In a 1997 New Zealand study (Durie, Allan, & Cunningham), the connection between cultural and community engagement and health was assessed.

The assessment of health and well-being among the elder population was based on Maori health perspectives and also took into account the importance of Elders in Maori society (a role and function that is similar to that of the elders in Aboriginal populations). In total, 400 Maori participants over the age of 60 years participated. The research found that: "in addition to economic and social considerations, well-being for older Maori was therefore conceptualized as an interaction between personal health perspectives and participation in certain key elements of Maori society e.g. land, language, marae (tribal gathering places)" (Durie, et al., 1997). Taking this information further, the study reported that Maori elders that ranked lowest on the "cultural index scale" (i.e. those less involved or less able to fulfill their cultural role) were also the most likely to have poor health; this was the case even for individuals that had similar basic standards of health and environmental circumstances. As such, the researchers concluded that: "a Maori view of well-being is closely linked to an ability to fulfill a cultural role. Measures of well-being that do not capture cultural identity will not be able to convey the nature of wellbeing, as it applies to Maori" (Dion Stout & Kipling, 2003; Durie, et al., 1997). This connects to and builds on the understanding of health developed throughout this book; that health is more than one's ability to avoid disease and reach specific measures, but that it also depends on broader socioeconomic factors that influence one's emotional, spiritual, mental, and economical well-being.

As this section shows, the risks associated with chronic disease development increase with age, due to the accumulation of risks across the life stages. Therefore, adulthood becomes an arena where chronic disease management becomes paramount and issues related to support systems and cultural practices become evermore important; this is especially true in vulnerable populations, such as the Aboriginal population. In preparing for this, it is important that the public health system design support services and education programs for the elderly so that diseases can be managed and accumulated risks can be held off. The health experiences of the eldest population viewed through a life course perspective helps us to understand the necessity of focusing on prevention and health promotion at the earliest stages of life and continuing this vigilance throughout life.

Part III: The Burden of Chronic Disease in Aboriginal peoples of Canada

1. Introduction

According to international indicators of health, Canadians' health status is among the highest in the world. In spite of this, the well-being of the Aboriginal population is comparable to that of many developing nations (Cooke, Beavon, & McHardy, 2004). This is exemplified by the increasing impact of chronic diseases on Aboriginal morbidity and mortality: while the impact of communicable diseases has declined in importance among Aboriginal populations, chronic diseases have emerged and grown into a significant health problem (Smeja & Brassard, 2000). Past and present studies have proven that Aboriginal Peoples in Canada bear a disproportionately higher burden of some chronic illnesses than do non-Aboriginal Canadians; almost one-third of Aboriginal people over the age of 15 report that they have been told by a health practitioner that they have a chronic health condition (MacMillan, et al., 1996). For example, in 2000/01, 60.1% of the off-reserve Aboriginal population versus 49.6% of the non-Aboriginal population reported having at least one chronic condition (Tjepkema, 2002). Of particular concern are statistics that show a high prevalence of many of the core chronic diseases. The burden of disease and disease trends among Aboriginal populations will be explored for the six core chronic diseases or disease groups: (1) diabetes, (2) cardiovascular disease, (3) chronic respiratory diseases, (4) musculoskeletal conditions, (5) cancer, and (6) severe mental illness. In addition to this, the impact of chronic diseases on one's mental health will be reviewed.

2. The Burden of Diabetes in Aboriginal peoples

2.1 Definition of Diabetes and Impaired Glucose Tolerance

Diabetes is one of the most reported on and documented chronic diseases in Aboriginal health because of its recent status as an 'epidemic' among Aboriginal Canadians. The discussion of diabetes, in an Aboriginal health context, largely refers to non-insulin dependent or type 2 diabetes mellitus. Type 2 diabetes is a metabolic disorder that is primarily characterized by insulin resistance, relative insulin deficiency, and hyperglycemia (i.e. elevated blood glucose). Type 2 diabetes is considered to be a chronic condition because once the body becomes resistant to insulin many of the resulting complications are ongoing. The problem with insulin resistance is that the body needs insulin to facilitate the entrance of glucose into cells in order to be used for energy. Without the transport of glucose into cells, it cannot be used and, instead, builds up in the blood. Excess glucose can cause damage to the body and, over time, can cause damage in the blood vessels and nerves, which increases the risk for eye, heart, blood vessel, nerve, and kidney disease (Burant & American Diabetes Association, 2004). The various acute and chronic complications associated with diabetes are what make it a considerable public health concern (Montour, Macaulay, & Adelson, 1989; Waldram, et al., 2006).

On a more moderate level, but with similar etiology and risk factors, is a condition called impaired glucose tolerance (IGT) or pre-diabetes mellitus. An individual has IGT when their blood glucose level is higher than normal, but not high enough to count as type 2 diabetes (Matthews, 2003). This is why the labels pre-diabetes, borderline diabetes, or chemical diabetes, are often used synonymously with IGT. The major concern with IGT is its potential to develop into full-blown type 2 diabetes. Because of this association, type 2 diabetes and IGT will both be discussed in this chapter with focus on the current prevalence of these conditions in the Aboriginal population in Canada and consideration of what these prevalence rates may mean for the future of Aboriginal health.

2.2 Burden of Type 2 Diabetes in Aboriginal peoples

Diabetes is considered to be a 'new' disease in the Aboriginal population that has increased rapidly in its magnitude and extent. For instance, it is only in the last 50 years that type 2 diabetes has been detected in Aboriginal populations in Canada (Health Canada, 2000b; T. K. Young, Reading, Elias, & O'Neil, 2000). A steady increase in the incidence and prevalence of type 2 diabetes in Aboriginal communities has caused researchers, policy-makers, and Aboriginal communities themselves to label type 2 diabetes as an epidemic among Aboriginal peoples. In addition to direct concerns about the prevalence of the two diseases, its disease management and the need for adequate prevention programs, there is concern about its severe complications and relation to other chronic diseases (T. K. Young, Reading,

Elias, & O'Neil, 2000). Such complications affect the circulatory system, eyes, kidneys, periodontal and nervous systems, and may result in premature mortality, disability, and compromised quality of life. A study done in Manitoba projected the future magnitude of this problem and the cause for such concern: it estimated that between 1996 and 2016, due to diabetes alone, there will be a 10-fold increase in the rate of cardiovascular disease; a 5-fold increase in strokes; 10 times as many dialysis starts; 10 times the rate of lower extremity amputations; and 5 times the rate of blindness among Aboriginal peoples (Greene, Blanchard, & Wajda, 1999).

2.2.1 Prevalence of Diabetes in First Nations, Métis, and Inuit Communities

As the prevalence of diabetes has been found to vary according to ancestry, language group, cultural area, and geographic location (Delisle, Rivard, & Ekoe, 1995), many of the studies conducted on diabetes in Aboriginal populations are specific to a particular community, nation, tribal council, Aboriginal population, or province. As a result, the 1991 Aboriginal Peoples Survey (APS) is the only national data available that reports on the prevalence of diabetes in First Nations, Métis, and Inuit populations (Waldram, et al., 2006). According to the APS' self-reported diabetes data, the prevalence of diabetes is lower in Inuit populations than it is in First Nations and Métis populations (S. G. Bruce, Kliewer, Young, Mayer, & Wajda, 2003).

The extent of the geographic variation in the prevalence of diabetes in Aboriginal populations is evident in a study conducted by Young, Szathmary, Evers, and Wheatley (1990), which mapped the cases of diagnosed diabetes among Aboriginal Canadians. They found that the lowest rates of diabetes were in the Northwest Territories while the highest were in the Maritimes (T. K. Young, Szathmary, Evers, & Wheatley, 1990). They also demonstrated that the prevalence of diabetes in Aboriginal peoples was higher (about 2-5 times higher) than their non-Aboriginal counterparts in all provinces and territories except British Columbia, the Yukon and the Northwest Territories (T. K. Young, et al., 1990). Overall, the prevalence of diabetes is also thought to vary along a north-south gradient: diabetes is generally lower in the North and higher in the South. This corresponds with data that reports Inuit people as having a lower prevalence of diabetes (~2%) (Bobet, 1998; First Nations Centre, 2005). This lower prevalence among Inuit and other Northern Aboriginal communities is often attributed to their more remote and isolated living situation. However, genetic susceptibility and environmental factors are other commonly cited explanations (Waldram, et al., 2006).

As the North comes into greater contact with the South and major urban centres, Inuit communities are thought to be at greater risk for contracting 'Western' diseases, such as diabetes (Bobet, 1997; Bruce, 2000a, 2000b; Greene, et al., 1999; Hegele, et al., 1999; McIntyre & Shah, 1986; Montour, et al., 1989; T. K. Young, Reading, et al., 2000). The reality of this risk has been shown in the rapidly rising rates of diabetes among Inuit peoples (I. P. Anderson, 2004; T. K. Young, Moffatt, & O'Neil, 1993): the prevalence of diabetes among the Labrador Inuit has climbed from 1.9% of the population in 1991 to 4% in 1999 (First Nations and Inuit Regional Health Survey National Steering Committee, 1999). These recent changes support the argument that geographic isolation, later contact with European settlers, and a sustained traditional way of life, were protective factors for Northern Aboriginal communities.

Although diabetes is a rising problem in the Inuit population, it has been more consistently reported as a chronic health concern for the First Nations population. However, the actual size and magnitude of the problem is still unclear. For example, the APS reported that the crude prevalence for diabetes in First Nations people was 6.4% and 8.5% for those living on- and off-reserve respectively (Bobet, 1998). In contrast, the 2002/2003 RHS reported an age-standardized prevalence of 19.7% for First Nations people. When limited to those 55 years of age or older, the rate increased to 35% (First Nations Centre, 2005). Similarly, one in four on-reserve First Nations people over the age of 45 were reported as living with diabetes (First Nations Centre, 2004). What these later RHS numbers suggest is that the prevalence of diabetes among First Nations people may have increased since 1991. Reports from Manitoba, which are based on information gained from the provincial database on hospitalizations and physician visits, supports this hypothesis: a rising trend in diabetes prevalence can be observed since the 1990s among First Nations people (Green, Blanchard, et al., 2003).

While it has been documented that diabetes is a concern for all First Nations, it is important to reiterate regional and community variations. Regional or community data can provide more context-specific information and demonstrate the various dimensions of the problem. For instance, a study conducted among the Oji-Cree reported a shockingly high prevalence

(40%) of type 2 diabetes and IGT; this represented the highest prevalence rate of any subpopulation in the world and is five times that of the Canadian average (Harris, Gittelsohn, et al., 1997).

Much less is known about diabetes among Métis peoples, but rates are comparable to, or lower than, the rate in First Nations for most age-sex groups (S. G. Bruce, et al., 2003). The national data, however, suggests that diabetes is generally higher among First Nations and Métis populations than the Inuit and the general Canadian population. While a smaller increase and a lower prevalence rate have been documented in the Métis population, the numbers are still higher than the national average: the crude prevalence of diabetes among Métis people was 5.5% in 1991, compared to 3.1% for the non- Métis population. According to the Métis National Council, the rate of diabetes among the Métis population as of 2006 is 5.9% (Métis National Council, 2006).

2.2.2 Gender stratification

In 1997, the rates of self-reported diabetes among First Nations men and women were reported to be, respectively, 3.6 and 5.3 times higher than among their age-sex matched non-Aboriginal counterparts (First Nations Centre, 2004). While these differences demonstrate, once again, the divide between diabetes in Aboriginal and non-Aboriginal populations, they also point to the stratification of diabetes according to gender. Because this gender difference adds important information to the burden of diabetes among Aboriginal peoples, relevant literature will be reviewed here.

In a study of two Algonquin communities in north-eastern Quebec (Delisle, et al., 1995) and the Oji-Cree community of Sandy Lake in north-western Ontario (Harris, Caulfield, Sugamori, Whalen, & Henning, 1997), the prevalence of type 2 diabetes was reported to be as high as 80% among women aged 50 to 64 years. Figures reported on national data show that women represent roughly 2/3 of the First Nations people who are diagnosed with diabetes (Bobet, 1997); in the general Canadian population, the reverse is true, where diabetes prevalence is generally reported to be higher among males than females (Health Canada, 1999). In addition to experiencing an overall higher prevalence of type 2 diabetes, many Aboriginal women have been diagnosed with gestational diabetes mellitus (GDM) (Mohamed & Dooley, 1998).

GDM is defined medically as any degree of glucose intolerance experienced with the onset of pregnancy or that which is first recognized during pregnancy (Matthews, 2003). Some glucose tolerance is known to deteriorate in all pregnant women as a result of the physiological and hormonal changes that accompany pregnancy (Hod, 2003). And, in the Western world, the deterioration of glucose tolerance reaches a sufficient level to fulfill the diagnostic criteria for gestational diabetes in approximately 2-3% of pregnancies (Whitaker, Pepe, Seidel, Wright, & Knopp, 1998). Surveys in Northern Quebec and Ontario have suggested that gestational diabetes may affect as many as 13% of pregnancies among Aboriginal women (Godwin, Muirhead, Huynh, Helt, & Grimmer, 1999; Harris, Caulfield, et al., 1997; Rodrigues, Robinson, & Gray-Donald, 1999). It has been suggested that difficulties with the documentation of the prevalence rates for gestational diabetes might be contributing to the high rates of GDM observed in many Aboriginal communities: for example, the first-time diagnosis of type 2 diabetes during pregnancy, and not etiologic GDM, is counted within the numbers. However, some research has shown that just under half of all pregnancies in women 35 years and older are associated with either pre-existing type 2 diabetes or gestational diabetes (Harris, Gittelsohn, et al., 1997). This information raises serious concerns about diabetes among Aboriginal women.

The prevalence rates, risk factors and outcomes of GDM between Aboriginal and non-Aboriginal women were directly compared for the first time in a Saskatchewan study (Dyck, Klomp, Tan, Turnell, & Boctor, 2002). This study reported that among residents within the Saskatoon District Health (SDH) region, the one-year prevalence rates for GDM were 3.7% for non-Aboriginal women and 6.4% for Aboriginal women. For residents outside the SDH, GDM prevalence rates were 3.1% for non-Aboriginal women and 22.8% for Aboriginal women (Dyck, et al., 2002). The greatest concern with GDM and maternal experiences of, or risks for, diabetes is the persistence of the disease beyond the woman's gestational period. For instance, a study in the Sioux Lookout Zone, reported that 70% of women diagnosed with GDM developed overt diabetes within three years (Mohamed & Dooley, 1998). This suggests a pressing need to target women's health and diabetes in Aboriginal communities.

2.2.3 The Childhood Burden of Diabetes

An increased prevalence of diabetes among a higher proportion of the younger Aboriginal population and an exaggerated prevalence of the early onset of diabetes in Aboriginal populations is a concern for Aboriginal children and youth. For example, a study documenting diabetes rates among the Haida Gwaii in British Columbia noted that 17% of adults age 35+ have type 2 diabetes (Grams, et al., 1996). Comparisons between First Nations communities and the non-First Nations population show that more than half (53%) of First Nations people living in First Nations communities with diabetes are 40 years or younger and 65% are less than 45 years (First Nations and Inuit Regional Health Survey National Steering Committee, 1999). As evident in the traditional label of adult onset diabetes, type 2 diabetes has typically not been observed in youth (Health Canada, 2000c). New cases in First Nations children, such as those detected among children as young as 5 to 8 years of age in the Island Lake region of north-eastern Manitoba (Dean, Mundy, & Moffatt, 1992) and in Northern Ontario (Harris, Perkins, & Whalen-Brough, 1996) put this label into question. In addition, screening for diabetes in a remote Northern Ojibwa-Cree community using fasting plasma glucose levels, found a high prevalence rate (3.6%) among females aged 10 to19 years (H. Dean, 1998; H. Dean, Young, Flett, & Wood-Steiman, 1998).

In general, Aboriginal peoples are younger than the non-Aboriginal population at the time of diagnosis and the onset of complications, and suffer greater disease severity at diagnosis (Goulet, et al., 2006; Ho, Gittelsohn, Harris, & Ford, 2006; Meatherall, et al., 2005; Pohar & Johnson, 2007; Simpson, Corabian, Jacobs, & Johnson, 2003). Despite their younger age Aboriginal people also suffer from higher mortality rates, higher complication rates, higher hospitalization rates, and longer hospital stays (Goulet, et al., 2006; Pohar & Johnson, 2007; Simpson, et al., 2003). This causes grave concern for the health and well-being of future generations.

2.3 Understanding the Numbers Now and in the Future

The statistics available on diabetes among Aboriginal peoples tell us that the distribution of diabetes among Aboriginal peoples varies markedly according to gender, geographical area, language group, culture area, latitude, longitude, and degree of isolation (Boston, et al., 1997; Health

Canada, 2000b; Jin, Martin, & Sarin, 2002; Macaulay, et al., 2003; Travers, 1995; T. K. Young, Reading, et al., 2000; T. K. Young, et al., 1990). In general, the prevalence is higher in the South than in the North, higher among women than men, higher among the less educated, and higher among urban and acculturated Aboriginal peoples (Bruce, et al., 2003; Daniel, Gamble, Henderson, & Burgess, 1995; Health Canada, 2005b; Jin, et al., 2002; Travers, 1995; T. K. Young, et al., 1990; Zimmet, Dowse, Finch, Serjeantson, & King, 1990). Despite what can be learnt from these numbers, a reliance on the number of reported diabetes diagnoses to determine prevalence rates can be questioned in terms of its reliability: because the onset of diabetes occurs an average 4-7 years before diagnosis, those currently diagnosed do not represent the total burden of disease (First Nations Centre, 2005; McKinlay & Marceau, 2000; T. K. Young, Reading, et al., 2000). For example, in Manitoba, undiagnosed diabetes constitutes approximately one-third of all cases of diabetes (S. G. Bruce, et al., 2003), and across Canada, the actual number of diabetics is probably two to three times greater (Health Canada, 2000b).

Further, because diabetes is developing earlier and at higher rates in the Aboriginal population, the impact of this disease on the health of the next generations is worrisome. It has been postulated, for example, that if these trends remain unchanged that the number of Aboriginal people with diabetes will triple by the year 2016 (Jin, Martin, & Sarin, 2002). An examination of the risk factors that occur across the life stages earlier in this book demonstrated the multi-faceted etiology of this disease and its interactions with other chronic diseases and chronic risk factors. Discussions of the ongoing need for research, effective health promotion strategies, interventions, and programs are also present later in earlier sections of this book.

3. The Burden of Cardiovascular Disease in Aboriginal peoples

3.1 Definition and Description of Cardiovascular Disease

Cardiovascular disease (CVD) has been noted to have the largest economic burden of any illness on Canada's health care (Health Canada, 2003a, 2005b; Lidgren, 2003). Since the 1960s, CVD has been decreasing in North America (Dorner & Rieder, 2004): much of the reduction in incidence and mortality has been attributed to lifestyle changes and behaviour modification, such as improving one's diet, exercising more frequently, and quitting smoking (Sytkowski, et al., 1996). Despite such changes, CVD remains the leading cause of death in most Western countries (Dorner & Rieder, 2004). The economic, social, and personal health burdens related to CVD in Canada, therefore, make it an important chronic disease to discuss and examine with regards to its impact on Aboriginal populations.

In an attempt to combat the current Canadian health crisis, a steering committee was created to develop the Canadian Heart Health Strategy and Action Plan (CHHS-AP) to set ambitious health targets for 2020 and produce recommendations for reaching those targets. One such target is to "end the CV[D] health crisis among Aboriginal/Indigenous peoples" by reducing the health burden of CVD on the Aboriginal population to parity with all other Canadians. Recommendations for achieving this target include: taking a partnership approach involving Aboriginal communities and government; creating a national Aboriginal Centre for chronic disease prevention and management; and helping Aboriginal peoples lead healthier lives through culturally appropriate means (Committee, 2009).

One must be careful when discussing CVD, as it is not just one disease. In fact, CVD refers to a heterogeneous class of diseases that concern the heart and/or circulatory system (Waldram, et al., 2006). The most common type of CVD is ischemic heart disease (IHD), also referred to as coronary heart disease, or coronary artery disease. IHD is a condition in which fatty deposits accumulate in the cells lining the walls of the coronary arteries, which serve as the heart's main blood supply. When fatty deposits gradually build up in the coronary arteries, the arteries become hard and narrow from atherosclerosis. Ischemia, which is a decreased supply of oxygenated blood to the heart muscle, develops from these conditions and can cause permanent damage to the heart. Complete blockage of the coronary arteries will lead to a heart attack (i.e. myocardial infarction) (Ontario Program for Optimal Therapeutics, 2000). While populations undergoing the transition from high to low rates of infectious diseases, such as Aboriginal peoples, tend to experience decreasing rates of diseases such as rheumatic heart disease, which is caused by infection, they also tend to experience increasing rates of IHD, which results from lifestyle and socioeconomic changes. Despite the interest in IHD, its causes, and its risk factors, data are often only available on CVD as a whole (Waldram, et al., 2006). As such, this section will discuss the general prevalence of CVD and, wherever possible, refer to ischemic heart disease (IHD).

3.2 Burden of Cardiovascular Disease in Aboriginal peoples

While there has been a documented decline in IHD prevalence across the Western world (Dorner & Rieder, 2004), such a decline has not been observed in certain subgroups of the population, such as Aboriginal peoples. Traditionally, Aboriginal peoples have experienced a low prevalence of IHD when compared to their non-Aboriginal counterparts. However, recent political, social and economic changes experienced by many Aboriginal communities have resulted in significant nutritional and lifestyle changes, such as a more calorie-dense and sedentary lifestyle, (Anand, et al., 2001) that have contributed to an increase in IHD prevalence (Anand, et al., 2001; Shah, Hux, & Zinman, 2000; Yusuf, Reddy, Ounpuu, & Anand, 2001).

Higher rates of IHD in Aboriginal populations were first documented in national studies of mortality among First Nations communities in the 1970s and 1980s (Waldram, et al., 2006). These studies found, however, that the rate of IHD was higher in females, but not in males (Mao, Moloughney, Semenciw, & Morrison, 1992; Mao, Morrison, Semenciw, & Wigle, 1986). In 1999-2000, the age-standardized mortality rate (ASMR) for all cardiovascular diseases was found to be slightly higher, but not a statistically significant difference, among First Nations people than it was among the non-First Nations population (Health Canada, 2003c; Waldram, et al., 2006). An increase in IHD prevalence among Aboriginal peoples, however, was definitely documented in a study conducted among 41 First Nations communities in Ontario (Shah, Hux, & Zinman, 2000). This study demonstrated that provincial hospital admission rates for IHD had more than doubled among the 41 First Nations communities – from 76 per 10,000 persons in 1984 to 186 per 10,000 in 1995 – while declining for the rest of the province (Harris, et al., 2002; Shah, et al., 2000). Among Sandy Lake residents, admission to hospital for IHD increased from a rate of 34.8 per 10,000 to 109.1 per 10,000 in 15 years (Harris, et al., 2002). A parallel trend was found in the admission rates for acute myocardial infarction (AMI or heart attacks) (Shah, et al., 2000). Further, AMI rates among First Nations are about 20% higher than the Canadian rate (First Nations and Inuit Health Branch, 2000/2001).

Data from 1981 to 1997 demonstrated that hospitalizations for illnesses relating to circulatory disease more than doubled for First Nations population in Ontario during this time period (Shah, et al., 2000), suggesting that circulatory disease has been increasing in importance as a major cause of morbidity. This hypothesis was corroborated when results from the 1997 RHS found that heart disease is 3 times higher and hypertension 2.5 times higher among First Nations/Inuit than among the general Canadian population (First Nations Centre, 2004). Further still, statistics from the 2002/03 RHS, which documented self-reported heart conditions in First Nations communities, reported a prevalence slightly higher than that of the Canadian population (7.6% vs. 5.6%). When controlled for specific age groups, First Nations adults were well above the Canadian average: First Nations adults 50 to 59 years of age had a prevalence of self-reported heart disease of 11.5% compared to 5.5% for the general Canadian population (First Nations Centre, 2005). While these statistics show that IHD poses an increasing threat for First Nations communities in Canada, the prevalence of CVD and specifically IHD in other Aboriginal communities is limited (Métis) and inconclusive (Inuit).

The challenge with understanding IHD in Arctic Native groups is that reports are conflicting. It has long been recognized and reported that IHD rates are lower than those of the non-Native population (Bjerregaard & Dyerberg, 1988; Middaugh, 1990; Waldram, et al., 2006; T. K. Young, Moffatt, & O'Neil, 1993). The reasoning for these low rates compared to First Nations is often attributed to the typically remote location of Aboriginal communities: their traditional marine diet and way of life are often thought to have acted as protective factors (Dewailly, et al., 2001). The reliability of the mortality statistics and other data used for these studies, however, has been questioned (Bjerregaard, Young, & Hegele, 2003). It is more accurate to say, therefore, that evidence documenting rates of CVD in Northern and Inuit communities is inconclusive. Bjerregaard, Young, and Hegele (2003) go on to say that there is a need to reassess the data on CVD in Inuit populations and re-evaluate the potential protective factors that a traditional diet can provide against rapid westernization and its related health risks.

As the concerns with Inuit CVD statistics demonstrate, and as is the case with all Aboriginal health issues, there are important regional and intertribal differences in CVD risk factors and disease rates. While the Inuit and Métis populations are important populations to target for future research, so too is the urban Aboriginal community (Yusuf, Reddy, Ounpuu, & Anand, 2001).

This is because most of the current data on CVD come from Aboriginal peoples living on-reserve and, therefore, very little is known about the burden of disease among the off-reserve population (Yusuf, et al., 2001). Therefore, studies that target all subsets of the Aboriginal population will be necessary to better understand the burden of cardiovascular disease among the Aboriginal population in Canada.

4. The Burden of Chronic Respiratory Diseases in Aboriginal peoples

4.1 Definition and Description of Chronic Respiratory Diseases

For this review, "chronic respiratory diseases" refers to any recurrent or persistent respiratory ailment related to the upper and/or lower respiratory system (i.e. the airways and other structures of the lung). Commonly cited chronic respiratory diseases are: asthma, chronic obstructive pulmonary disease (COPD), respiratory allergies, occupational lung diseases, chronic respiratory tract infections, tuberculosis, and pulmonary hypertension (WHO, 2008b).

In order to engage in a productive discussion of chronic respiratory tract infections in the Aboriginal population, this section will focus on five key conditions discussed in the literature, which pose a significant current or potential impact on the health and well-being of Aboriginal peoples. They are: (1) tuberculosis, (2) chronic otitis media, (3) chronic/recurring respiratory tract infections, (4) COPD and (5) asthma. First, however, a brief overview of chronic respiratory disease in Aboriginal populations is provided below.

4.2 General Burden of Chronic Respiratory Disease in Aboriginal peoples

Although chronic respiratory conditions are traditionally uncommon in First Nations communities (Sin, Wells, Svenson, & Man, 2002), Aboriginal peoples are adversely (and increasingly) affected by respiratory disease when compared with their non-Aboriginal counterparts (Mao, et al., 1984; Mao, et al., 1992; Mao, et al., 1986; Morrison, Semenciw, Mao, & Wigle, 1986; T. K. Young, 1983). For instance, the Aboriginal population is at an increased risk of death from respiratory diseases and experience an excess of morbidity (Fraser-Lee & Hessel, 1994). The risks for and burden of respiratory disease is especially profound for Aboriginal children: 13 out of 20 respondents in a survey of Native children's health ranked respiratory illness as the most serious child health concern (Petersen, Singleton, & Leonard, 2003). A prospective study of children born in 1973 in Canada's North reported that respiratory illness accounted for 36% of infant deaths and was the leading cause of infant mortality (Orr, McDonald, Milley, & Brown, 2001). This statistic is compounded by the fact that infant mortality rate among Aboriginal peoples is double the Canadian average (Sin, et al., 2002). For these reasons, we consider chronic respiratory conditions an important disease to include in this book's discussion. This is also why a significant number of the articles, reports, and documents reviewed in this chapter will draw from child and youth studies.

4.3 Tuberculosis

Tuberculosis (TB) is a chronic bacterial infection that is spread through the air and usually infects the lungs (U.S. National Library of Medicine and the National Institutes of Health, 2005). Tuberculosis is classified as a chronic disease because individuals with TB remain infected for life. Since the development of treatment (antibiotics) and prevention (vaccines) for this disease, TB is largely thought to be a concern of the past. Unfortunately, this is far from the truth: about 2 million people die from this treatable (Health Canada, 2002) disease each year (Skeiky & Sadoff, 2006; WHO, 2005b). Not surprisingly, TB infection and mortality is most common in developing nations, where poverty, poor (or no) access to health care, and inadequate living conditions persist (WHO, 2005b). For similar reasons, Aboriginal peoples are still fighting this disease (PHAC, 2004). As TB is the leading cause of death in HIV/AIDS-infected individuals (Grange, Story, & Zumla, 2001; Skeiky & Sadoff, 2006) and HIV/AIDS is a serious and increasing concern within the Aboriginal population (First Nations and Inuit Regional Health Survey National Steering Committee, 1999; Ring & Brown, 2002; Spittal, et al., 2002), the interactions between HIV/AIDS and TB, as well as their independent health risks, should continue to be of focus and interest for future research (Health Canada, 2002).

4.3.1 Adult Burden of Disease

Tuberculosis among Aboriginal peoples reached epidemic proportions following their contact with European settlers, which began in the 16th century and carried on until the 20th century (Hoeppner & Marciniuk, 2000). The Public Health Agency of Canada (PHAC) has reported that

TB incidence continues to follow patterns of colonization, which run on a gradient from south to north: tuberculosis rates are highest in the prairie provinces and the North, where contact with Europeans occurred after Aboriginal communities located in more Southern regions (PHAC, 2004). Since the Aboriginal population was infected with TB later than the non-Aboriginal population, it is not entirely surprising that Aboriginal people continue to suffer a higher burden of this disease (Gaudette & Ellis, 1993; Wang, Noertjojo, Elwood, & FitzGerald, 2000). What is surprising is the increased disparity between the prevalence of TB in Aboriginal and non-Aboriginal populations.

Since the beginning of the 20th century, tuberculosis rates have fallen dramatically in Canada, and they continue to decrease today (PHAC, 2004; Wang, et al., 2000). However, rates of TB infection within the Aboriginal population have not seen as significant a decline (Wang, et al., 2000) and are now considerably higher than the Canadian average (T. K. Young & Casson, 1988). In 1970, the Aboriginal rate was twelve times higher than the non-Aboriginal rate, with 212 cases per 100,000 population compared with 17; by 1995, the Aboriginal rate was thirty-nine times higher, with 70 per 100,000 population cases versus 1.8 (Hoeppner & Marciniuk, 2000). In order to get a more accurate reading of the prevalence of TB in Aboriginal populations, data obtained by Health Canada between 1990 and 2000 was controlled for ethnicity. With such a control, it was demonstrated that Aboriginal incidence rates rise from 8-10 times to 20-30 times the Canadian-born, non-Aboriginal average (Health Canada, 2002).

These and other statistics documenting the high burden of disease in the Aboriginal population indicates that tuberculosis will be an ongoing concern for the future (Smeja & Brassard, 2000). In 1999, 16% of new active and relapsed TB cases that were reported to the Canadian Tuberculosis Reporting System were from the Aboriginal population (PHAC, 2004). This number is disproportionately high considering that Aboriginal people only make up 3.7% of the Canadian population (Statistics Canada, 2008a). The fact that 92% of the Aboriginal cases were new active cases causes even more concern for the persistence and presence of the disease (Health Canada, 2002). The significantly younger age of Aboriginal people with TB, as compared with their non-Aboriginal counterparts, is also concerning for the future. The burden of TB experienced by Aboriginal children and youth is further discussed on next page.

4.3.2 Child and Youth Burden of Disease

In 2002, Health Canada reported that young Aboriginal adults (15-34 years of age) have the highest proportion of infectious tuberculosis cases and are at the greatest risk of contracting the disease. In addition to high youth rates, paediatric cases of TB in 1999 were observed to be 29 times higher in Aboriginal populations than in the non-Aboriginal population. Although this reflects a decreased rate of infection from previous years (Health Canada, 2002), the critical numbers emphasize the magnitude of its impact on the younger generations.

A brief plateau in the rate of TB infection occurred during the 1980s; this was an anomaly to a decreasing trend occurring in the 20th century. In response to the sustained prevalence of TB in Canada in the 1980s, newborns were routinely vaccinated with bacilli Calmette-Guerin (BCG). Since this time, the BCG has become the world's most widely used vaccine, despite evidence of variable efficacy (0-80%). Data from animal and human trials indicate that variances are related to pre-existing immune responses to antigens that are common to environmental mycobacterium and mycobacterium TB (Andersen & Doherty, 2005). In Cree communities, BCG has been administered since 1982[7] (Smeja & Brassard, 2000). The efficacy of BCG in preventing pulmonary TB is still unknown, but meta-analyses suggest that its efficacy in preventing serious forms of TB in children can be up to 80% successful (Colditz, et al., 1995). The absence of active TB and TB meningitis diagnoses among Cree infants since 1980 also provides some evidence for the protective effects of the BCG vaccination (Smeja & Brassard, 2000). However, current thinking on the BCG vaccine is that it should only be administered to newborns with the highest risk, which includes many Aboriginal infants and those with HIV positive mothers (Colditz, et al., 1995; Menzies, Tannenbaum, & FitzGerald, 1999).

4.4 Chronic Otitis Media

Otitis media is an inflammation or infection of the middle ear, which occurs when the Eustachian tube (the passage from the throat to the middle ear) is blocked (U.S. National Library of Medicine and the National Institutes of Health, 2005). This condition can be chronic or acute, suppurative

---

7 From 1982 to 1989, BCG was repeated at age one if the child's annual tuberculin skin test (TST) was less than 5 mm; since 1989, BCG has only been given to children at birth.

or secretory (Med-Help, 2004). This review will focus on chronic otitis media, as its purpose is to study chronic respiratory problems in Aboriginal peoples. Since chronic suppurative otitis media is the most common form of infection, this is what chronic otitis media refers to in the rest of the document. While otitis media is not usually included in discussions of chronic respiratory diseases, it is related to the under-recognized area of chronic bacterial respiratory infections (P. S. Morris, 1998). It is specifically included here because of its prevalence in the Aboriginal population and because it is important to study it in the context of its respiratory etiology.

Chronic otitis media occurs when the Eustachian tube is repeatedly blocked or remains blocked for long periods of time; this may be the result of a lingering acute ear infection or persistent ear infections (U.S. National Library of Medicine and the National Institutes of Health, 2005). Prolonged or repeated infections can permanently damage the ear and cause partial or complete deafness (Med-Help, 2004; U.S. National Library of Medicine and the National Institutes of Health, 2005). Since ear infections are most common in children, chronic otitis media usually develops at a young age and persists into adulthood (Med-Help, 2004), causing considerable damage to the ear throughout the life cycle.

Chronic suppurative otitis media (CSOM) is uncommon in most developed countries, which is why it is often descried as a disease of poverty (Coates, Morris, Leach, & Couzos, 2002). The WHO has defined a prevalence of 4% or greater for CSOM as a "massive public health problem" (WHO, 1998). In many Aboriginal communities and populations in circumpolar regions (Martin & Macdonald, 1998), the proportion of children with CSOM is ten times the WHO's cut-off (Coates, et al., 2002). In response to a high prevalence of otitis media among Indigenous peoples in North America in the 1960s, a mandatory notification program for severe cases of otitis media was introduced. A program to ensure continued surveillance of the disease is needed today (P. S. Morris, 1998) since otitis media is endemic among Northern Inuit, First Nations, and Métis children: prevalence rates for these communities are sometimes reported to be as much as 40 times those found in non-Aboriginal urban communities (Bowd, 2005).

Much of the research on otitis media in Aboriginal populations has been done in Australia. Although there are obvious geographic and cultural differences between Canada's and Australia's Indigenous populations, strong parallels can be drawn between their health status: Aboriginal peoples bear a disproportionate burden of this disease comparable to their Australian counterparts (Coates, et al., 2002), which is why trends from Australia have relevance for Indigenous peoples. In order to exemplify the prevalence of this disease in Aboriginal communities, a review of some important Australian studies is provided below. In the future, similar studies should be done in Canada in order to develop accurate and useful Aboriginal statistics.

In Australia, severe otitis media in rural Aboriginal children is part of the spectrum of chronic bacterial infections of the respiratory tract that burdens this population (Leach, 1999; Leach & Morris, 2001; P. S. Morris, 1998). The high rates of CSOM demonstrate the absolute burden on Australian Aboriginal health: 95% of Aboriginal children observed had otitis media, versus 30% of non-Aboriginal children (Boswell & Nienhuys, 1996).

The situation is even worse in rural and remote regions, where this chronic disease affects almost every child. In one rural Aboriginal community, all infants under three months of age were diagnosed with acute otitis media; a follow-up study indicated that the situation had not resolved itself by early childhood, as 60% of the cases developed into chronic otitis media (Leach, 1999). The long term impacts of this disease is further exemplified by a study in the Northern Rivers Area (a region in New South Wales, Australia), where among 61.08% of the children studied had middle ear problems of some type, 10.8% had unilateral hearing loss and 22.16% had bilateral hearing loss (Thorne, 2003). Since extremely high resultant rates of conductive hearing loss (>50%) were often attributed to this population's poor classroom success (Leach, 1999), this disease presents considerable physiological and sociological problems and challenges for the community.

Furthermore, Australia's National Trachoma and Eye Health Program highlighted the prevalence comorbidity of this disease among its Aboriginal population (Moran, Waterford, Hollows, & Jones, 1979): otitis media was the most common bacterial respiratory disease diagnosed by health officials and was associated with extremely high rates of pneumonia, meningitis, and bronchiectasis in the Aboriginal population (Gandevia, 1967; Hanna & Torzillo, 1991; Maxwell, 1972; Torzillo, et al., 1995; Torzillo, Waterford, Hollows, & Jones, 1983). A similar association was documented for Indigenous people in Papua New Guinea, where early infections in the nasopharynx and high rates of pneumonia were linked to a high prevalence of otitis media (Gratten, et al., 1986; Montgomery, et al., 1990).

Despite the lessons that can be learned from Australia's research in this area, it is important to consider the particularities of the burden of chronic otitis media among the Aboriginal population. This means developing targeted, focussed studies to assess the incidence, prevalence, and overall burden of the disease.

4.5 Chronic/Recurring Respiratory Tract Infections

An acute respiratory tract infection (Jacono, Jacono, Cano, Segami, & Rubin, 1996) can affect one or both of the upper and lower respiratory systems and can be a short-lived, persistent, or recurrent condition. The most common respiratory tract infections are bronchitis, bronchiolitis, pneumonia, pneumonitis, and croup (Kurzius-Spencer, Wind, Van Sickle, Martinez, & Wright, 2005).

For reasons largely unknown, Aboriginal children tend to have an increased risk of developing respiratory tract infections (Evers, Orchard, & McCracken, 1985; Harris, et al., 1998; Orr, McDonald, Milley, & Brown, 2001; Sin, Wells, Svenson, & Man, 2002): over 90% of native children studied experienced a lower respiratory infection[8] within their first year of life. Although no comparison to a Caucasian population was given in this study (Petersen, Singleton, & Leonard, 2003), other studies demonstrate that Aboriginal children have greater respiratory concerns than their non-Aboriginal counterparts. For example, Evers et al. (Evers, et al., 1985; Evers & Rand, 1982, 1983), who extensively examined the impact of acute respiratory infections (ARIs) on Aboriginal and non-Aboriginal populations in south-Western Ontario, found that despite the affluence of the Aboriginal communities studied[9], the incidence of lower respiratory disease among First Nations children was almost three times that of the non-Aboriginal population (Evers, et al., 1985). A population-based study of infants and young children in north-western Ontario documented similar findings: respiratory tract infections were reported to be the main cause of illness in this population, and Aboriginals were more likely to report respiratory conditions than the non-Aboriginal children studied (Harris, et al., 1998). More specifically, the incidence of pneumonia has been reported to be 17 to 18 times greater for native children under the age of two than for non-native children (Evers & Rand, 1982, 1983). As Inuit populations in Canada

8 "Lower respiratory tract infection" refers to bronchitis, bronchiolitis, or pneumonia.

9 The communities studied were reported as having much higher living standards and greater access to medical care than other Aboriginal regions in Canada.

demonstrate similar trends for lower respiratory problems, it is reasonable to assume that all of Canada's Aboriginal peoples experience a high risk of upper and lower respiratory tract infections (Fraser-Lee & Hessel, 1994; Koch, et al., 2003).

The prevalence of ARIs in Aboriginal children is worrisome because these infections have the potential to develop into chronic conditions: respiratory infections weaken the pulmonary system, which can cause permanent lung damage and lead to the development of chronic conditions (Anto, Vermeire, Vestbo, & Sunyer, 2001). The risk of Aboriginal peoples developing chronic respiratory conditions from ARIs is evidenced by the tendency for Status Indian children to have multiple episodes of pneumonia and bronchitis (Fraser-Lee & Hessel, 1994). Within the first two years of life, Aboriginal children experience repetitive bouts of pneumonias, bronchiolitis, and are routinely hospitalized for respiratory complications. Although these often improve after the age of two, recurrent wheezing and chronic coughing has been shown to continue throughout life (Petersen, et al., 2003). Evidence for a link between infections and chronic disease was reported in a recent study of Alaskan natives, when 40% of the children studied showed signs of respiratory infections and chronic respiratory disease (Lewis, et al., 2004). A study of young Indigenous children in New Guinea made similar observations: a significant relationship was found between the presence of early respiratory infections and the subsequent onset of asthma (H. R. Anderson, 1978).

4.6 Chronic Obstructive Pulmonary Disease (COPD) and Asthma

Chronic obstructive pulmonary disease (COPD) is identified by a patient's "shortness of breath, cough, and sputum production"; its long-lasting course is characterized by an irreversible decline of forced expiratory volume in one second (FEV1), increasing presence of dyspnoea and other respiratory symptoms, and a progressive deterioration of health status (Cardinal, et al., 2004). COPD's broad impact on the respiratory system means that it often overlaps with other respiratory conditions, such as chronic bronchitis, emphysema, and asthma that share common symptoms and have co-morbid interactions. Nonetheless, this respiratory problem, alone, has been noted as a leading cause of mortality and disability world-wide: approximately 5-15% of adults in industrialized countries have COPD, and the numbers continue to grow. In 1990, COPD was the twelfth known cause of combined mortality and disability world-wide: by 2020, it is expected to rank fifth (Anto, et al., 2001). As such, this disease will require comprehensive hospital and community health services in Canada.

Asthma shares many similar symptoms, risk factors, and treatment methods with COPD (Anto, et al., 2001), which is why they are often grouped together. However, it is important to identify them as separate chronic diseases. By definition, "asthma is a chronic health disorder characterized by symptoms of cough, shortness of breath, chest tightness, and wheeze" (Cardinal, et al., 2004). Asthma is the most common chronic disease afflicting children today (Lewis, et al., 2004), and the prospects of this disease are not promising: childhood asthma is increasing in prevalence and severity, especially among children 5 years of age and younger (Woolcock & Peat, 1997). Historically, asthma has not affected Aboriginal peoples, but its increasing prevalence in Aboriginal populations today demonstrates that these communities are becoming very vulnerable to the disease (Downs, Marks, Belosouva, & Peat, 2001; Liu, et al., 2000; Sin, et al., 2002).

The prevalence of asthma in Canada's Aboriginal population has been progressively explored since Houston et al. (1979) reported a high prevalence of chronic cough and bronchial wall thickening among native children, as compared to white children, in Northern Saskatchewan (Kurzius-Spencer, Wind, Van Sickle, Martinez, & Wright, 2005). Recent studies of Aboriginal peoples have shown that Aboriginal peoples are considerably burdened by asthma (Lewis, et al., 2004; Liu, et al., 2000; Sin, et al., 2002): Aboriginal children in their first year of life have rates of hospitalization for asthma and bronchiolitis that are two to three times the rate of non-Aboriginal children (Lewis, et al., 2004; Liu, et al., 2000). In connection with asthma, native children have also reported higher hospitalization rates than non-native children for wheezing and breathing problems (Liu, et al., 2000; Sin, et al., 2002).

Within Canada, Aboriginal-specific research will be needed to create new policies and programs aimed at reducing the burden of COPD and asthma, since studies on Aboriginal peoples report that this population is 2.1 times (95% CI 2.0, 2.2) and 1.6 times (95% CI: 1.6, 1.6) more likely to have an emergency hospital appointment and office visit for asthma or COPD, respectively, as compared with their age-matched, sex-matched non-Aboriginal counterparts. The fact that Aboriginal people were also 55% (95% CI: 52, 58) less likely to see a specialist and 66% (95% CI: 63, 70) less likely to undergo spirometry for these conditions than non-Aboriginal people (Sin, et al., 2002) raises significant concern about the adequacy of health services and health policies in Canada.

5. The Burden of Musculoskeletal Conditions in Aboriginal peoples

5.1 Definition and Description of Musculoskeletal Disease and Disorders

Musculoskeletal diseases and disorders have been identified as the most common cause of severe pain and disability. As a result, they place a massive burden on societies and health care systems around the world (Lidgren, 2003). In Canada, musculoskeletal diseases and disorders account for 10.3% of the total economic burden of illness: second only to cardiovascular diseases (Health Canada, 2003a, 2005a; Lidgren, 2003). The economic burden of these diseases is only expected to increase as the Canadian population increases (Lidgren, 2003). As such, musculoskeletal conditions are a timely and relevant topic to discuss. The incidence and prevalence of these diseases in Aboriginal populations is important to consider, as the Aboriginal population also ages and as chronic diseases become a more prominent feature of Aboriginal health.

In order to begin to examine and discuss the burden of musculoskeletal diseases and disorders in Aboriginal populations, it is important to be clear as to what this title encompasses. Classification of musculoskeletal diseases and disorders has changed over time, making it difficult to determine the availability and reliability of information and certain diseases and disorders (Jacobson, De Groot, & Samson, 1994). For example, according to a 1989 WHO report, there were over 100 diseases and disorders of the musculoskeletal system, which were referred to as 'rheumatic diseases' and characterized by inflammation of the connective tissues, especially the muscles, joints, and associated structures (Encyclopædia Britannica, 2006; WHO, 1989). However, the modern disease classification (ICD-10) does not include such term as 'rheumatic diseases;' instead, musculoskeletal diseases and disorders are classified according to the affected organ (ICD-10. International Classification of Diseases, 2006). Alternatively, some researchers use the 1958 ACR (formerly, the American Rheumatism Association) criteria in their studies, while others used 1987 ACR criteria. While still debated it seems that the term "musculoskeletal diseases and disorders" includes nearly 150 different diseases and disorders (Lidgren, 2003).

Out of these many diseases and disorders, arthritis is the most common and most prevalent. At its most basic level, arthritis means inflammation of the joints: 'arth' meaning joint, 'itis' meaning inflammation. It would be overly simplistic, however, to assume that arthritis is one condition when, in fact, there are a number of different types of arthritis (Canadian Arthritis Society, 2004). Two of the most common arthritic conditions are rheumatoid arthritis and osteoarthritis (Canadian Arthritis Society, 2004; Health Canada, 2003a). Other common types of arthritis discussed in the literature include: spondiloarthropathies and arthropathies associated with systemic lupus erythematosus and gout (Health Canada, 2003a). While there are many different types of arthritis, much of the literature reports on the prevalence of musculoskeletal conditions using the general heading "arthritis/rheumatism:" this label is used to refer to the collection of painful joint disorders that range from those related to wear and tear of cartilage (e.g. osteoarthritis) to those associated with inflammation resulting from an immune disorder (e.g. rheumatoid arthritis). Because of this often dual reference, it is often difficult to separate these two conditions. As such, an examination of the burden of arthritis is based on general information about chronic arthritic conditions (including rheumatoid arthritis). The specific burden of rheumatoid arthritis, however, will not be discussed separate from the general discussion of arthritis, as its etiology is largely unknown and because it is likely a result of infection is largely considered to be preventable and not predisposed to risk factors across the life course. More general understandings of arthritis as a preventable condition make this general term more appropriate to discuss, as is the specific burden of osteoarthritis. In addition to the general burden of arthritis and osteoarthritis, osteoporosis will be discussed. Osteoporosis is often discussed in tandem with arthritis because it is also a condition of the bones. Rather than the characteristic inflammation and joint damage of arthritis, osteoporosis is characterized by very low bone mass that leads to an increased risk of traumatic or low impact fractures (Dictionary, 2002b; ICD-10, 2006).

5.2 Burden of Arthritis in Aboriginal peoples

In the general Canadian population, arthritis is one of the most prevalent chronic conditions in Canada and the number one cause of disability and health care utilization (B. C. Canada, 2001; Health Canada, 2003a; WHO, 1989). Arthritis has also been cited as the most common chronic condition in Canada's Aboriginal population (B. C. Canada, 2001; Canadian Arthritis Society, 2004; First Nations Centre, 2005; Health Canada, 2003a; John, Hagan Hennessy, & Kerby, 2000). For example, a study conducted in British Columbia found that arthritis was more common among Aboriginal people (17%) than in the non-Aboriginal population (5%) (B. C. Canada, 2001). Likewise, prevalence of self-reported arthritis is also higher in the American Indian, Eskimo and Aleut populations (17.5%), compared with of US White population (15.2 %) (Lawrence, et al., 1998). In Manitoba, it was found that twice as many First Nations Manitobans were diagnosed by a physician for rheumatoid arthritis, degenerative arthritis and other non-descript forms of arthritis, compared to non-Aboriginal Manitobans (Barnabe, Elias, Bartlett, Roos, & Peschken, 2008). As arthritis involves damage to the joints of the body, it is not surprising that this condition tends to increase with age. The significant increase in the distribution of arthritis among First Nations adults according to age is exemplified in the figure below (First Nations Centre, 2005).

Figure 1. Prevalence of arthritis among First Nations adults by age group (total age adjusted)

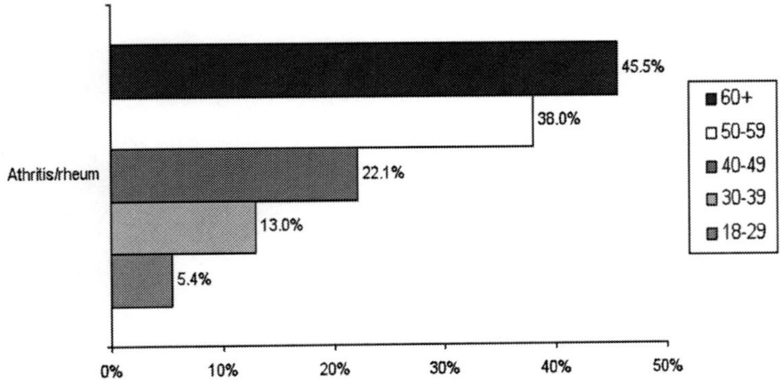

Source: (First Nations Centre, 2005).

Arthritis has also been documented to vary across gender lines, with women being disproportionately represented. Arthritis is particularly high among older Aboriginal women: 70% of Aboriginal women aged 65 and older, compared with 50% of their Canadian counterparts, were diagnosed with arthritis (Canadian Arthritis Society, 2004). While these statistics are based on comparisons between the Canadian population and on-reserve Aboriginal women, similar trends in arthritis prevalence are found within the urban, off-reserve Aboriginal population (Health Canada, 2003a). Variances in arthritis prevalence according to gender and ethnicity are exemplified in the figure below.

Figure 2. Self-reported prevalence of arthritis among Aboriginal people living off-reserve and non-Aboriginals, by age and sex

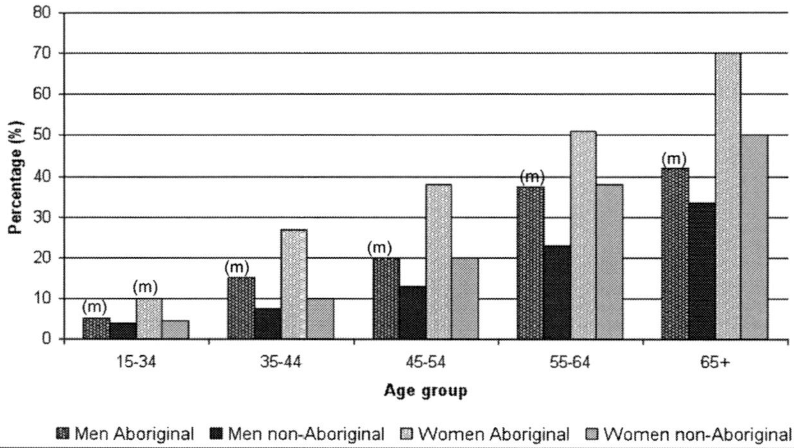

Source: (Health Canada, 2003a).

Note: Differences between Aboriginals living off-reserve and non-Aboriginals are statistically significant at $p < 0.05$ for females of all age groups and for males aged 35 to 44. (m) indicates that the coefficient of variation is between 16.6% and 33.3%.

While the information and statistics presented above help paint a picture of the burden of arthritis in Aboriginal populations, a brief discussion of osteoarthritis is included here to highlight the specific burden of this type of arthritis in Aboriginal populations and to help lead into a discussion of osteoporosis.

5.2.1 Osteoarthritis

Osteoarthritis (OA), also known as arthrosis, degenerative arthritis, degenerative joint disease, and the "wear and tear" arthritis, is the most common form of arthritis. It is caused by a breakdown in the cartilage, which covers and acts as a cushion inside joints, and destruction or decrease of synovial fluid that lubricates those joints. While osteoarthritis can affect any joint, it usually affects the peripheral joints (i.e. hips, knees, hands and spine) (Dictionary, 2002a). While osteoarthritis is thought to be largely hereditary, aging joints, previous injuries, and obesity are thought to exacerbate risk.

As noted above, OA is the most common type of arthritis, affecting 10% of Canadian adults (Health Canada, 2003a). While the literature on OA is limited in Aboriginal populations, Thommasen (2006) has noted that rural Canadians and rural Aboriginals are the most vulnerable for OA (H. V. Thommasen & Zhang, 2006). Earlier studies (1960-61) of OA in North American Native populations found that 68% of Blackfoot Indians, 65% of Pima Indians, and 24% of Alaska Eskimos had OA of the hands. These rates are particularly high considering that the same study showed that 7-12% of the White populations with OA in 1968 (Peschken & Esdaile, 1999). A 1986 study, however, reported much lower OA prevalence rates for Inuit men (1%) and Inuit women (2%) (Peschken & Esdaile, 1999). Gender specific prevalence of hip OA was found to be similar in Aboriginal and non-Aboriginal populations, being less than 10 % in all age and gender groups (Hirsch, et al., 1998). In Australian Aborigines, OA appears to be particularly common in the temporomandibular joints, right elbow and knees (Roberts & Roberts-Thomson, 1999).

As this data only provides a superficial view of the burden of osteoarthritis in Aboriginal populations, it will be worthwhile to engage with the mainstream arthritis literature and examine the prevalence and risk for arthritis, and particularly osteoarthritis, in Aboriginal populations.

5.3 Osteoporosis

Osteoporosis is defined and diagnosed by the WHO in women as a bone mineral density (BMD) 2.5 standard deviations below peak bone mass (20-year-old healthy female average) as measured by Dual energy X-ray absorptiometry (Leslie, et al., 2006; Lewiecki & Silverman, 2006; Nicholas & Chen, 2002; WHO, 1994). While this testing is commonly used, some researchers have voiced doubts about the accuracy of osteoporosis diagnosis among children, men and women of other ethnic groups when based on the WHO criteria (Nicholas & Chen, 2002). The term "established osteoporosis" is used to refer to the increased presence of fragility fractures (WHO, 1994).

Overall, the data on osteoporosis in Aboriginal populations is limited. The most available studies of osteoporosis related to and report on fracture rates, without data on or reference to mean BMD values. As such, it is difficult to estimate whether elevated fracture rates in these populations are related to osteoporosis or to other factors, such as high risk activities, falls due to age, qualitative changes in bone structure, and variability in bone geometry (Nicholas & Chen, 2002). Keeping these other potential fracture factors in mind, a recent retrospective, population-based, matched cohort study of fracture rates in Manitoba's Aboriginal and non-Aboriginal populations has reported higher rates of hip, wrist and spine fractures in Aboriginal versus. non-Aboriginal population (Leslie, et al., 2006). This data is provided in the table below.

Table 1. Fracture rates in Aboriginal and non-Aboriginal Manitoba adults (age 20 years and older), 1984-2003

Fracture site	Aboriginals	Non-Aboriginals
Hip	1.1 %	0.6 %
Wrist	1.3 %	0.5 %
Spine	1.6 %	0.9 %

Source: (Leslie, 2006).

As there is not a lot of information on osteoporosis in Aboriginal population, future studies are warranted to unpack the underlying burden of this disease among Aboriginal peoples. The potential for higher rates of osteoporosis due to linkages with other chronic diseases and risk factors in Aboriginal populations, such as obesity and diet, make this an important area for future research.

6. The Burden of Cancer in Aboriginal peoples

6.1 Definition and Description of Cancer

Normally, the human body is made up of billions of cells that develop in predictable ways. Cancer is caused when those cells begin to develop unpredictably: it is characterised by uncontrolled growth and spread of abnormal cells in the body (PHAC). Cancer is not one disease, but is a group of more than 100 different and distinctive diseases. Cancer can involve any tissue of the body and have many different forms in each body area. Most cancers are named for the type of cell or organ in which they first develop. Cancerous cells are most often detected when they begin to lump together and form a mass, commonly known as a tumour. As the tumour grows, it may damage and/or takeover nearby tissue and metastasize (spread) into another part of the body (Canadian Cancer Society, 2008). Documentation of cancer mortality and incidence rates largely indicate that cancer is less prevalent among Aboriginal people than it is among the non-Aboriginal population (Waldram, et al., 2006). Because determining the exact prevalence of cancer in Aboriginal populations is a challenging task, the reliability and accuracy of the current statistical data is limited (First Nations and Inuit Regional Health Survey National Steering Committee, 1999). Taking this into consideration, this section will begin by outlining several of the surveillance methods used to examine cancer in Aboriginal populations. A presentation of the current data on cancer prevalence will follow this discussion.

6.2 Cancer Surveillance in Aboriginal peoples

All Canadian provinces are equipped with population-based cancer registries that report data on the number of cancer cases within their population (Waldram, et al., 2006). The challenge with determining the incidence and prevalence of cancer in Aboriginal populations is that most of these provincial registries do not report cancer data by ethnicity (First Nations and Inuit Regional Health Survey National Steering Committee, 1999). Further, Statistics Canada does not compile or report on cancer data by ethnic status (Waldram, et al., 2006).

Nevertheless, there are several surveillance methods that are used to study cancer in Aboriginal populations. These methods include: gathering information using residence codes for reserves; using First Nations indicators in health insurance numbers; using the ethnicity recorded on death certificates; or through linking the data with the Federal Department of Indian Affairs Status Verification System. The problem with these surveillance methods, however, is that they can include inappropriate individuals or exclude appropriate individuals in the registry, thus, producing biased results (L.D. Marrett, Jones, & Wishart, 2004). For example: the use of residence codes may include non-Aboriginal people living on reserve, exclude urban Aboriginals and other off-reserve Aboriginals, and also exclude individuals who may have had to leave their home community to receive treatment (Rosenberg & Martel, 1998). The use of provincial health card numbers is troublesome because not all health card numbers have First Nations indicators. Finally, death certificate ethnicity data is often inaccurately recorded and the Status Verification System is not always up to date (L.D. Marrett, et al., 2004). Due to these concerns, other methods of studying disease burden in Aboriginal populations would be beneficial, as would creating specific Aboriginal cancer registries regionally and/or nationally.

A specific registry that has been established is a Canadian Inuit cancer registry comprised of cases from the Northwest Territories, Nunavik, and Labrador. This unique registry was developed as part of an international circumpolar review of cancer among Inuit populations (Gaudette, et al., 1996). While the Northwest Territories and Nunavut both have current cancer registries, this collaborative Inuit registry does not undergo maintenance or updating (Waldram, et al., 2006).

Consequently, data on the burden of cancer in Aboriginal populations is obtained by developing linkages between ethnicity and provincial registries. National data is obtained by linking the provincial data together. While there are problems with this reporting system and data sources, it is important to review the information gained through them. Prior to a discussion of the burden of cancer in Aboriginal populations, it is important to explain that in addition to a faulty registry system, very few Canadian studies that have been published to date are restricted in their generalizability and validity beyond the very source of the information. Such other limitations are summarized well by Marrett & Chaudhry (2003):

> The limitations include small numbers of cancers, different methods of identifying cancers in [First Nations] people versus the general populations groups, numerators and denominators derived from different sources, lack of currency in terms of the years studied, and restricted populations (for example, only those on reserves). Further, few have had the numbers and length of study period to be able to examine changes in cancer patters over time.

Taking these limitations into account and the fact that there are only a handful of studies on cancer incidence and mortality published in Canada (L. D. Marrett & Chaudhry, 2003), the following section will try and summarize the general information on the burden of cancer in Aboriginal populations.

6.3 Burden of Cancer in Aboriginal peoples

While there are only a few studies on the burden of cancer in Aboriginal populations, the vast majority of them focus on First Nations people (L. D.

Marrett & Chaudhry, 2003). Information has also been documented on the Inuit population (Gaudette, Gao, Freitag, & Wideman, 1993; Nielsen, Storm, Gaudette, & Lanier, 1996) and even less specifically focused on the Métis population (Kliewer, Mayer, & Wajda, 2002). Because of the differences in the amount of literature and the burden of disease among the three different Aboriginal groups, they will be reviewed separately below.

6.3.1 Burden of Cancer among Canada's First Nations population

Data collected in the 1970's from British Columbia (Gallagher & Elwood, 1979), north-western Ontario (T. K. Young & Frank, 1983), and Manitoba (T. K. Young & Choi, 1985) all reported lower incidence rates for First Nations people when all cancer sites were combined (Waldram, et al., 2006). However, a study by Rosenberg and Martel (1998) that examined time-trend from 1972-76 and 1987-91 noted that cancer incidence and mortality appear to be increasing on reserves. They found that while cancer incidence has been traditionally lower in First Nations populations, cancer incidence and pattern of survival were found to be similar to that of the non-First Nations population, except for a higher proportion of cases and mortality caused by cervical and gallbladder cancer in females and kidney cancer in both sexes (Rosenberg & Martel, 1998). Marrett and Chaudhry (2003) reported similar trends in their study of cancer incidence and mortality among Ontario First Nations people between 1968 and 1991. They reported that cancer incidence was significantly lower in Status Indians, compared to the general population, for some of the most common cancers (e.g. breast, lung, prostate, and colorectal). Despite these comparatively lower rates, the incidence rates for all types of cancer increased significantly over the time periods of the study. Other less common cancers, such as cervical, gallbladder, and kidney, were exceptions to this trend: cancer of the gallbladder is twice as common in Status Indian men and women than it is in the general population; cervical cancer is 1.73 times higher in Status Indians than in the general population and is the second most common cancer in Indian women; and, kidney cancer appears to occur more frequently in Status Indian populations, but the rate for both sexes was not statistically significant (L. D. Marrett & Chaudhry, 2003). This and other key information gathered in Marret and Chaudhry's (2003) study and its comparison with the other major studies conduced in provinces across the country are summarized in the table on the following page.

Table 2. Cancer incidence, prevalence, and mortality in Ontario, Manitoba, Saskatchewan, and British Columbia

Province	Related Literature	Cancer incidence, prevalence, and mortality
Ontario	(Marrett & Chaudhry, 2003; Young & Frank, 1983)	Incidence of kidney, mouth, throat and stomach cancers is similar in Aboriginal and non-Aboriginal populations for both sexes; Incidence of colorectal cancer is equivalent in Aboriginal and non-Aboriginal male populations; Incidence is increasing in Aboriginal populations for the leading cancers, such as breast, prostate, lung and colorectal, and is approaching overall Ontario cancer rates; Incidence for cervical cancer is declining in female Aboriginal populations, and is approaching the Ontario rate for women; Survival rates are significantly lower in Aboriginal populations, compared to the non-Aboriginal population, for all cancers combined, for prostate cancer in Aboriginal men, and for breast cancer in Aboriginal women; Survival rates are similar in Aboriginal and non-Aboriginal populations for other leading cancers (lung, colorectal and cervix).
Manitoba	(Young & Choi, 1985)	Aboriginal women have higher incidence of cervical cancer than non-Aboriginal women; The incidence rate of kidney cancer is higher in the Aboriginal population.
Saskatchewan	(Gillis et al., 1991)	Survival for breast cancer is poorer in the Northern Aboriginal population than in the Southern non-Aboriginal
British Columbia	Threlfall et al, 1986	Aboriginal women have a higher incidence of cervical cancer than non-Aboriginal women; Pancreas and stomach cancer incidence rates in the Aboriginal population is similar to that of the BC population; Survival rates for all cancers combined is similar in both Aboriginal and non-Aboriginal populations.

Source: (L. D. Marrett & Chaudhry, 2003).

As this table shows, the amount and type of information available in each province varies greatly.

In an attempt to get a national perspective, the leading cancer mortality rates in on-reserve First Nations and the general Canadian population were compared by Statistics Canada in 2000 and 2001. These analyses found that First Nations cancer mortality rates, except for male prostate cancer, were lower than those for the overall Canadian population (Statistics Canada, 2001d). This is demonstrated in the figure below.

Figure 3. Selected Mortality Rates, First Nations On-Reserve and Canada

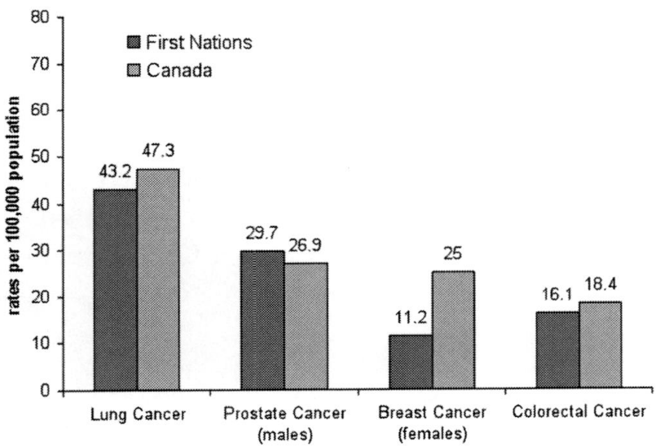

Source: (Statistics Canada, 2001d).

While these lower rates are encouraging, the literature reviewed above indicates that cancer rates are increasing in First Nations populations and are quickly approaching cancer rates in the non-First Nations population (L. D. Marrett & Chaudhry, 2003).

6.3.2 Burden of Cancer among Canada's Inuit population

The burden of disease among Canada's Inuit population is quite different from that noted among First Nations. For example, it has been reported that Inuit people are at a high risk for several rare cancers, including nasopharyngeal, salivary gland, and esophageal cancer (Gaudette, et al., 1993; Waldram, et al., 2006). Since the 1970's, however, these "traditional Inuit cancers" (Waldram, et al., 2006) have declined, while more common cancers among the non-Inuit population, such as lung, cervical, colon, and breast cancers, have increased (Hildes & Schaefer, 1984; Schaefer, Hildes, Medd, & Cameron, 1975).

Cancer data collected during the time period of 1969-1988 from Greenland, Canada and Alaska provide important insights into the study of cancer patterns among Circumpolar Inuit populations. For instance, the results of this international, collaborative study demonstrated that the age-standardized rates increased by 22% for Aboriginal men and 24% for Aboriginal women from 1969 to 1988, which did not deviate significantly from cancer rates observed in the mainstream populations of Canada, Denmark and Connecticut (USA) (Nielsen, Storm, Gaudette, & Lanier, 1996). However, significant differences between Inuit populations and the comparison populations were found in the site-specific cancer rates. Compared with the populations of Canada, Denmark and Connecticut (USA), the Inuit were found to be at higher risk of lung, nasopharynx, salivary glands, oesophagus, gallbladder and extrahepatic bile ducts cancers. Inuit males had a higher incidence rate for cancer of the liver and stomach, while Inuit females were at higher risk of cervical and renal cancer. The leading cancer sites in Circumpolar Inuit males and females are represented in Table 3 below.

Table 3. The Leading Cancer Sites in Circumpolar Inuit (1969-1988)

Rank	Male population		Female population	
1	Lung	28.3%	Cervix	17.6%
2	Colon	8.1%	Lung	13.7%
3	Stomach	7.0%	Breast	11.4%
4	Nasopharynx	6.5%	Colon	9.6%

Source: (Nielsen, et al., 1996).

While Circumpolar Inuit populations have reportedly high levels of certain cancers, they are also at lower risk for cancer of the bladder, breast, endometrium, prostate, as well as for lymphomas, Hodgkin's disease, leukemia, multiple myeloma and melanoma (Nielsen, et al., 1996). Investigations into the underlying reasons for differences in prevalence among the Inuit will be important to investigate in future research.

6.3.3 Burden of Cancer among Canada's Métis population

Very little information is available on the health status of Métis people in Canada, particularly with regards to cancer. In order to find ways to develop a pool of information on the burden of cancer among Manitoba's Métis population, the Manitoba Métis Federation (MMF) approached CancerCare Manitoba to discuss information sharing and develop a dataset (Kliewer, et al., 2002). As was discussed in the beginning of this section, databases maintained by provincial organizations do not have specific ethnic or racial indicators (First Nations and Inuit Regional Health Survey National Steering Committee, 1999). A pilot study done to assess the feasibility of linking a sample of the MMF membership list to Manitoba Health (the provincial database) and CancerCare Manitoba databases in order to retrieve more concrete information on the health status of Métis. As the data used to calculate the prevalence of cancer in this study consists of small numbers, it is not possible to report extensively on cancer site. It is possible, however, to discuss some preliminary observations about the burden of cancer among the Métis in Manitoba gained from this study (Kliewer, et al., 2002).

Out of the study sample, six (6) males and twenty (20) females were diagnosed with cancer in 1995-1997. Overall, this meant that the average annual age-standardized cancer incidence rate was lower for Métis men as compared to the general male Manitoban population. The incidence for Métis women was slightly higher than the general female Manitoban population. The rate of cervical cancer was found to be substantially higher among Métis women. The crude age-standardized prevalence rates for Métis women were lower for Métis women. When age-specific prevalence rates were taken into account, however, the prevalence was higher for Métis women than it was for all Manitoba women. The prevalence of malignant and other neoplasms were lower for Métis men than for the non-Métis population, while malignant neoplasms were higher in Métis women and other neoplasms were comparable to the general female Manitoba population. This overall high prevalence of cancer in Métis women is attributed to the substantially higher rates of cervical cancer as compared to Manitoban women. This comparable with studies of cervical cancer reported for Manitoba's Treaty Status Indians (T. K. Young, Kliewer, Blanchard, & Mayer, 2000).

While this brief discussion of cancer rates among the Métis in Manitoba begins to paint a picture of the burden of cancer among Métis peoples, its limitations as a pilot study and its provincial location highlight that further information and data is needed.

7. Burden of Severe Mental Illness in Aboriginal peoples

7.1 Definition and Description of Chronic Mental Illness

Mental illnesses have been defined as "states of distress that result from complex interactions between person and environment over the course of decades of individual development" (Spaudling, Sullivan, & Poland, 2003). Defining mental illnesses as 'chronic,' however, is an issue of much debate. This is largely because of questions about the meaning of the term 'chronicity.' For instance, does chronicity refer to the duration of symptoms, the functional disabilities that result from mental illness, or both? (Bachrach, 1988; Soreff, 1996) If both, are duration and disability equally important in determining chronicity? Further, is chronicity established after a specific duration of persistent illness or after a certain number of recurrent episodes? (Soreff, 1996) There is also a question of whether chronicity can be inferred from the diagnoses of particular mental disorders. Nevertheless, there is general agreement among researchers that diagnosis is "a necessary but not sufficient condition for defining chronic mental illness" (Bachrach, 1988).

The use of the word 'chronic' has also raised the concerns of mental health advocates who believe the term implies and perpetuates a sense of hopelessness with regards to the management and treatment of severe mental illnesses (Bachrach, 1988). Labelling an individual as chronically mentally ill can be perceived to limit that person to a continuous or life-long illness (Bachrach, 1988; Lefley, 1990; Soreff, 1996). To avoid the stigma associated with the word 'chronic', the phrase 'severe and persistent mental illness' or simply, severe mental illness (SMI) is more commonly used, and will be used here.

Despite the many challenges of defining SMI, some researchers have attempted the task. Stein (1995) defined SMIs as "those illnesses that are longer than one year in duration, cause significant dysfunction, and meet certain diagnostic criteria" and likewise, Rosenberg and colleagues (2005) defined SMI as "a diagnosis of a major mental illness, disability in important life spheres (e.g. school, work or family function), and persistence of illness and disability". Soreff (1996) provided a broader definition, that is, the "severe and persistent disabilities that result primarily from mental illness" and acknowledged the vast differences that exist in the duration of illness and degree of disability that influence diagnosis. Indeed, "those who might be defined as chronically mentally ill today vary widely in their diagnoses, their treatment histories, their functional levels, and their treatment needs" (Bachrach, 1988). Taking these differences into consideration will be important as we review the burden of severe mental illnesses in Aboriginal peoples. This is because the limited literature on mental illness in Aboriginal peoples and in limited contexts in which it has been examine can encourage an over-generalization of findings and present a limited perspective.

7.2 Burden of Severe Mental Illnesses in Aboriginal peoples

Although there is some disagreement over which mental disorders qualify as severe and persistent, schizophrenia, bipolar disorder and major depressive disorder are generally categorized as such (Bachrach, 1988; S. D. Rosenberg, Drake, Brunette, Wolford, & Marsh, 2005; Stein, 1995). Therefore, these disorders should be included in this discussion of the SMIs that affect Aboriginal individuals. Unfortunately, the limited research available on bipolar disorder among Aboriginal Peoples hinders our ability to discuss the topic. This shows, without a doubt that research in this area would be of value. Nonetheless, Aboriginal experiences of schizophrenia and major depressive disorder, as well as post-traumatic stress disorder and addiction, will be discussed below. While literature related to Canadian contexts is used wherever possible, a lack of specific studies on mental health in Aboriginal peoples means that studies from other Indigenous populations is used to supplement the Canadian material. As important lessons about prevalence, burden and treatment of SMIs can be learned from Canada's international counterparts, these discussions will be informative for the Canadian context.

7.2.1 Schizophrenia

Early studies of schizophrenia have indicated that there are differences in the incidence and expression of symptoms between Indigenous and non-Indigenous patients. For instance, Bates and van Dam (1984) found a much lower incidence of schizophrenia among First Nations of coastal British Columbia than the Caucasian population, though incidence rates were not equal across all First Nations groups. Mowry and colleagues (1994) noted that among persons diagnosed with schizophrenia in Western Australia, Australian patients varied significantly from non-Indigenous patients in the diagnostic symptoms reported in their medical records. The authors suggested a number of possible explanations for the differences, including: misinterpretation of symptoms by mental health professionals; bias in clinical examination and record keeping; unique manifestation of schizophrenia among Indigenous patients; or misdiagnosis of Indigenous patients suffering from alternative mental illnesses (Mowry, et al., 1994).

Recent research on schizophrenia in Indigenous populations is limited; however, the studies that do exist both contradict and support earlier research on the topic. Researchers in New Zealand reported Maori to be over-represented among adolescents who self-reported schizotypal symptoms (i.e. magical thinking, hallucinatory tendency, self-referential ideation, and perceptual aberration) (Linscott, Marie, Arnott, & Clark, 2006). Conversely, Robin and colleagues (2007) reported that for two North American Indian tribes, the prevalence of schizophrenia matched that expected for the non-Indigenous population, and among second-degree relatives of individuals with schizophrenia, the prevalence was lower than expected. The authors acknowledged that the prevalence rate of schizophrenia was not higher for these tribes despite the increased risk associated with the high prevalence of alcohol consumption, drug use and poor socioeconomic conditions within the tribal communities. They conclude that psychiatric misdiagnosis, reliance on small sample sizes, and limited cultural awareness have lead to over-estimation of the prevalence of schizophrenia among North American Indians (Robin, et al., 2007). Therefore, socio-cultural factors must be considered prior to making a diagnosis of schizophrenia (Robin, et al., 2007). Overall, it is clear that there is no prevalence rate of schizophrenia consistent across all Indigenous groups. When prevalence rates do differ from those of non-Indigenous populations, these differences may have less to do with biological differences and more to do with the diverse cultural influences of Indigenous peoples.

As the above discussion demonstrates, more targeted research on schizophrenia in the Canadian context is needed. Further, research into and discussion of treatment, potential interventions, and ways to improve the health and well-being of individuals living with schizophrenia would be beneficial.

7.2.2 Depression

There is some debate as to whether depression is a chronic illness or not (Gask, 2005; Parker, 2005; Van Weel-Baumgarten, 2005). 'Depression' and 'major depression' are terms that oversimplify and gloss over the multitude of causes, expressions, trajectories, and outcomes of the various depressive disorders that exist (Parker, 2005). Given the effect that a patient's history, help-seeking behaviour, social environment, and compliance can have on their response to treatment; as well as the influence of a health practitioner's skills, priorities, biases, and preferred treatment methods; it can be argued with reason that for some individuals the experience of depression is chronic and for others it is not (Van Weel-Baumgarten, 2005).

Depression is often assumed to be prevalent among Indigenous peoples because of high suicide rates in some communities (H.V. Thommasen, Baggaley, Thommasen, & Zhang, 2005); however, reports of depressive episodes among Indigenous peoples vary considerably. Further, reports of depression among Aboriginal peoples are almost exclusively restricted to First Nations, with little information for Métis, Inuit, and non-Status Natives (Health Canada, 2005a). Even the information we have on First Nations is largely self-reported in surveys and, therefore, only offers a crude estimate of depression rates with no information regarding specific mental disorders. In an effort to get a better understanding of the depression among Aboriginal peoples, this section will review the literature available in Canada and internationally. It is the hope of the authors that the lack of information available across the Aboriginal groups in Canada will encourage future research in this area and understanding of the variability of Aboriginal peoples and their health.

Data from the 2000/2001 Canadian Community Health Survey revealed that 13.2% of the Canadian off-reserve Aboriginal population had experienced a major depressive episode in the past year, a rate 1.8 times that of the non-Indigenous population; however, similar depressive rates were found between Indigenous and non-Indigenous peoples living in the Canadian territories as well as between those with high and low household incomes (Tjepkema, 2002). Another Canadian survey, the 2002/03 RHS, found that 30.1% of adult and 27.2% of youth First Nations respondents had felt sad, blue, or depressed for a period of two weeks or more in the year prior to the survey (First Nations Centre, 2005). Those respondents reported suicide ideation and attempts twice as often as respondents who did not feel sad, blue or depressed. Research conducted by the Government of Canada found that approximately 8% of Canadian adults experience major depression at some time in their lives (Health Canada, 2002) compared to 12% reported by First Nations in 2001 (Canada, 2006a). A comprehensive study of depression, anxiety and use of antidepressant medication in the Bella Coola Valley of British Columbia revealed that the prevalence rate of depression-anxiety disorders among Indigenous people was slightly lower, though not significantly different, than the prevalence rate among non-Indigenous people (H. V. Thommasen, et al., 2005). Other studies however have not found a statistically significant difference between Aboriginal and non-Aboriginal people in terms of depression rates (H. V. Thommasen, et al., 2005). In contrast, a study conducted in the United States, American Indians of Northern Plains and Southwest tribes were found to be at lower risk for 12-month and lifetime major depressive episodes than individuals sampled from the general population, though significant differences in risk were found between the two tribes and between men and women of the tribes (Beals, Novins, Spicer, Mitchell, & Manson, 2005). Among a sample of Navajo American Indians, 37% had experienced a major depressive episode in their lifetime, 11% reported current depressive disorders, and one-fifth (20%) had experienced depressive, anxiety and substance use disorders in their lifetime (Storck, Csordas, & Strauss, 2000). The variations that exist in the depressive experiences of Indigenous peoples suggest that, similar to the general population, depression will be chronic for some individuals and not others.

Some Canadian research has examined the manifestation of depression among Aboriginal peoples. Kirmayer, Fletcher et al. (1994) reported symptoms among the Inuit of Nunavik analogous to the ICD 10 diagnostic criteria for depressive episode including: wanting to be alone, refusing to talk with others, not eating, not sleeping, and crying a lot. Söchting, Corrado et al. (2007) suggested that the symptom picture among Aboriginal people seeking mental health services is often quite extreme in terms of impairment in interpersonal relations, poor self-image, inability to regulate and control intense negative emotions, and serious substance abuse (Söchting, Corrado, Cohen, Ley, & Brasfield, 2007). Some have suggested that the traditional means of coping with stress and psychological pain have changed in recent times to impulsive behaviour and substance abuse (Kirmayer, Fletcher,

Corin, & Boothroyd, 1994). Among Aboriginal men, many avoid medical health services and cope with their depression by drinking alcohol or hunting (Canada, 2006a; Kirmayer, et al., 1994). The use of alcohol as a means of dealing with trauma among Indigenous peoples is also explored in American research. Brave Heart (2003) identifies alcohol use as a way of avoiding painful feelings through self-medication. The important influence that alcohol and drug abuse has on one's mental health is evident in the figure below, which list the factors considered by First Nations living on reserve in Saskatchewan to be very important for maintaining mental health (First Nations Centre, 2004).

Figure 4. Factors considered very important in maintaining mental health

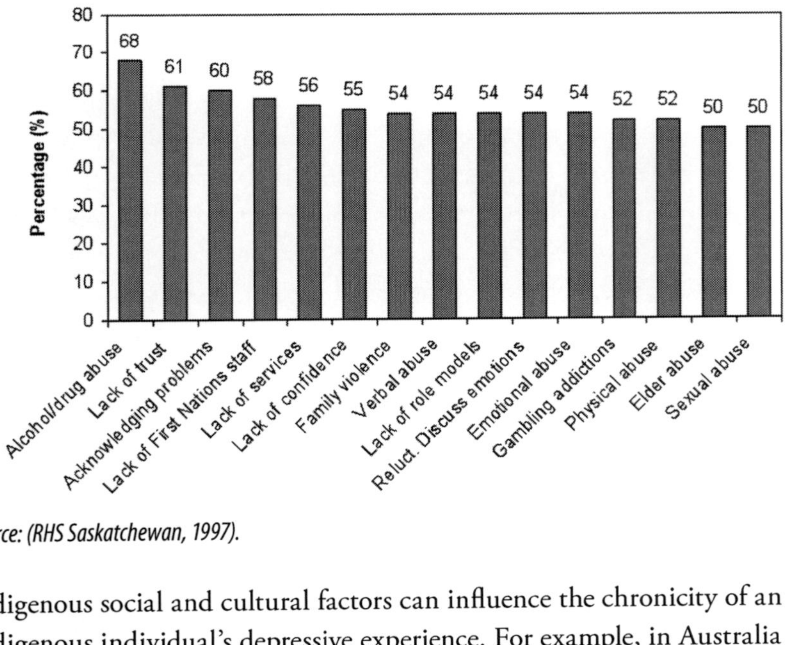

Source: (RHS Saskatchewan, 1997).

Indigenous social and cultural factors can influence the chronicity of an Indigenous individual's depressive experience. For example, in Australia where nearly three-quarters (72%) of an Indigenous sample indicated that depression was an inborn characteristic of an individual that could not be resolved through treatment, depressive experiences may be chronic more often than not (Vicary & Westerman, 2004). Yet in the United States, Navajo patients who described cultural causes and interpretations of their depressive experiences were able to reach remission (i.e. a sense of balance and well-being and reduction of depressive symptoms) through individualized, culturally-appropriate healing practices (Storck, et al., 2000).

Thus, not only is treatment "dependent upon the cultural explanation given to the illness" (Vicary & Westerman, 2004), but the outcome of the treatment is dependent upon culture as well. For instance, because of the evidence for non-medical means of coping with depression, depression rates estimated from service utilization data for Aboriginals are likely underestimates of the true prevalence of depression (Kirmayer, et al., 2000). Data from the 2002/03 RHS state that 71.7% of individuals feeling sad, blue or depressed ranked family and friends as their top choices of support. Only 9.1% and 8.4% ranked psychiatrist or psychologists as a support (First Nations Centre, 2005). More research is required in this area in order to ascertain how detection methods should be altered to make them more appropriate (Jackson-Triche, et al., 2000).

7.2.3 Post-Traumatic Stress Disorder

Post-traumatic stress disorder (PTSD) is a psychological disorder that arises from an individual's experience of trauma (Chansonneuve, 2007; Corrado, et al., 2003; Mitchell & Maracle, 2005). A diagnosis of PTSD requires the following symptoms to be present: re-experiencing the traumatic event (such as flashbacks or nightmares), avoidance of stimuli associated with the traumatic event, and increased physiological arousal (such as rapid breathing and increase heart rate). Affects on the mind, emotions, body, and spirit include: anxiety; intrusive thoughts and memories; sleep disturbances; angry outbursts; exaggerated startle response; and hyper-sensitivity. It is not uncommon for PTSD to exist in concurrence with additional mental and physical health problems such as depression, substance abuse, heart disease, and stomach problems (Corrado, et al., 2003; Mitchell & Maracle, 2005).

The availability of prevalence rates of PTSD among Aboriginal peoples, and even Indigenous peoples worldwide, is limited. The majority of research on PTSD in Indigenous populations sampled from adult American Indians of Southwest and Northern Plains tribes. Veterans of these tribes were more likely to qualify for diagnosis of lifetime and current PTSD than Caucasian veterans (Beals, et al., 2002). The prevalence of lifetime PTSD for adults of the Southwest tribe was 21.9%, and was higher for women (25.4%) than for men (17.9%) (Robin, Chester, Rasmussen, Jaranson, & Goldman, 1997). In the Northern Plains tribe, 15% of the sample met criteria for lifetime PTSD, and the participants who met PTSD criteria were more likely to be diagnosed with lifetime major depressive disorder and alcohol abuse than those who did not (Sawchuk, et al., 2005). The high prevalence rates of PTSD found among adults of these tribes were attributed to high rates of exposure to traumatic events and not to any increased vulnerability of American Indians to PTSD (Robin, et al., 1997; Sawchuk, et al., 2005). One research group found that among a sample of American Indian adolescents in substance abuse treatment, the proportion of participants that met criteria for PTSD (10.3%) was modest in comparison to the proportion that had traumatic experiences (98%) (Deters, Novins, Fickenscher, & Beals, 2006). The authors suggested that future research should explore the resiliencies that Indigenous youth develop in the face of repetitive traumas.

A minority of Indigenous survivors of the residential school system present diagnostic symptoms similar to those of post-traumatic stress disorder, while many others struggle with commonly associated symptoms, such as relationship difficulties, deficient parenting skills, little knowledge of Indigenous culture, reduced interest and participation in cultural activities, and alcohol or drug abuse associated with violent outbursts (Brasfield, 2001; Corrado, et al., 2003; Dion Stout & Kipling, 2003). The term 'residential school syndrome' is sometimes used to describe this group of symptoms, though the term remains controversial because specific diagnostic criteria has not yet been formally established (Brasfield, 2001). Furthermore, Chrisjohn and Young (1995) argue that a regular set of symptoms associated with attendance at residential schools is unlikely to exist due to the wide range of experiences and behaviours of residential school survivors. Research on PTSD among Indigenous groups should be regarded with similar caution, as the present symptoms are likely to vary significantly from individual to individual, as well as between Indigenous and non-Indigenous populations, as a result of unique histories, experiences and coping strategies.

7.2.4 Addiction

Much like other mental disorders, addiction lacks an established definition and clear diagnostic criteria. Sometimes, addiction is confused or used interchangeably with other terms, such as dependence or compulsion. For the purposes of this discussion, addiction is defined as "a process whereby a behaviour, that can function both to produce pleasure and to provide relief from internal discomfort, is employed in a pattern characterized by: (1) recurrent failure to control the behaviour (powerlessness) and (2) continuation of the behaviour despite significant negative consequences (unmanageability)". Addiction is not synonymous with dependence (gratification of needs) or compulsion (evasion or avoidance of internal discomfort), but instead involves both dependence and compulsion together (Goodman, 1990). Addictive behaviours may also include gambling, overeating, working, or using psychoactive substances

Although addiction to a psychoactive substance involves abuse of a substance, the abuse of a substance is not always addictive (National Native Addictions Partnership Foundation Inc., 2000). Often, substance abuse occurs infrequently or in an experimental setting; however, this pattern may not hold true for all populations. Research suggests that patterns of substance abuse differ between Indigenous and non-Indigenous populations (Beauchamp, et al., 2004; First Nations Centre, 2005; Fournier & Crey, 1997; Health Canada, 2003c; Saggers & Gray, 1998; H. V. Thommasen, Hanlon, Thommasen, & Zhang, 2006). Most studies of substance use among Indigenous populations have focused primarily on the use of tobacco and alcohol. It can be argued that tobacco abuse poses the greatest long-term consequences to Indigenous health, yet, for many Indigenous communities, the immediate health and social consequences of alcohol abuse are of primary concern (Saggers & Gray, 1998). As discussed earlier in this book, tobacco abuse is a major risk factor across the life course for many other chronic diseases. Here, the discussion of addiction will focus on alcohol addiction.

7.2.5 Alcohol Addiction

The disease model of alcoholism, which defines alcohol addiction as a chronic disease, is supported by many but regarded as limited by others. For example, Alcoholics Anonymous, which has wide-reaching influence on how alcohol addiction is viewed and treated, endorses the disease model of alcoholism. Many people have found comfort and social support through accepting this view of alcohol addiction, and have been successful in attaining and maintaining sobriety. Suissa (2003) has argued that the disease model is also supported by specific groups, including Irish and Indigenous groups, because it fits with their cultural understandings of alcohol and addiction. However, the 'all-or-nothing' orientation of the disease model, which when applied to alcohol addiction means an "individual is or is not an alcoholic forever" (Suissa, 2003), is limited by it applicability and treatment options. For instance, 'all-or-nothing' demands that alcoholics abstain from alcohol. Unfortunately, such a view can overlook the benefits to be gained from brief intervention and harm reduction strategies. In addition, 'all-or-nothing' cannot be applied universally across addictions; an individual addicted to overeating cannot abstain from eating, just as a workaholic cannot abstain from working. Thus, living with or overcoming addiction can sometimes require more than simply abstaining; addicted individuals may need to learn skills that facilitate healthy moderation instead (Goodman, 1990).

Nonetheless, abstinence has helped many alcohol addicted Indigenous individuals to achieve a healthy and well-balanced lifestyle. Much of the existing research on Indigenous alcohol use has found that abstinence and lower frequency of use are more common among Indigenous peoples than non-Indigenous people (First Nations Centre, 2005; Fournier & Crey, 1997; Saggers & Gray, 1998; H. V. Thommasen, et al., 2006). Often, a large portion of Indigenous abstainers are previous alcohol users (Saggers & Gray, 1998). Wardman and Quantz (2005) sampled from Indigenous peoples of Western Canada and found that most previous alcohol users described 'hitting rock bottom' before achieving abstinence. Often, binge drinking was used to numb the pain caused by physical and sexual abuse, low self-esteem, loss of culture and identity, and family history of substance abuse (Dennis Wardman & Quantz, 2005). Many of the individuals that were currently maintaining sobriety found strength through renewed spirituality and involvement in cultural traditions. In another study, narratives of Navajo men who previously drank but currently abstained from alcohol suggested that it was common for Navajo men to reach a point in life when issues of health, religion, family, and wealth took priority over alcohol use (Quintero, 2000). For these men, alcohol was associated with loss of tradition and an out-of-balance lifestyle. Often formal treatment was not sought, as the desire to return to traditional living was sufficient motivation to abstain.

Although the rate of abstinence is higher and frequency of alcohol use is lower, it is also the case that, binge drinking occurs more frequently among Indigenous than among non-Indigenous alcohol users. In other words, "those who do drink tend to drink heavily" (Canada, 2006b). It is likely this pattern of alcohol use that contributes to the alcohol-related problems experienced by Indigenous communities. This burden is exemplified by the fact that Alcohol was a factor in 6.4% of injuries incurred by First Nations youth and over one-quarter (27.1%) of assaults against First Nations youth (First Nations Centre, 2005). Rothe (2005) reported that within nine

First Nations communities, respondents considered alcohol abuse and drinking and driving to be "normal, community-endorsed behaviours". The proportion of Status Indian deaths that are alcohol-related is nearly one-quarter (23.5%) while drug-induced deaths account for 6.2% of Status Indian deaths (First Nations Centre, 2005). High rates of alcohol-related morbidity and mortality have also been reported in Australia (Saggers & Gray, 1998). Reasons given by Indigenous individuals for their alcohol use include boredom associated with living in a communities of limited recreational and employment opportunities and need to self-medicate to anesthetize the pain of poverty, racism and violence; thus, it is more likely community social and economic structure rather than individual or cultural values that contribute to the high prevalence of alcohol abuse in Indigenous communities (Rothe, 2005).

7.3 Burden of Severe Mental Illnesses on Community Health

Community health is influenced by physical and social environments (Smye & Mussell, 2001) of both the past and present (First Nations Centre, 2005). Dysfunction within family and community life has wide-ranging influence on mental health (Mussell, Cardiff, & White, 2004) and an individual's experience of mental health can impact their family and community. Conversely, therefore, correcting relationships within the family and facilitating community healing can promote health and wellness (Canada, 2006a; Warry, 1998). As such, the following section will focus on the potential influence of SMIs on communities and the community-wide burden of disease.

When a population is marginalized and culturally suppressed, the mental health of that population, whether Indigenous or not, is affected at the individual, family, and community levels (Canada, 2006a). Mental health problems often occur in the form of social burdens such as family violence, substance abuse and suicide (Canada, 2006a; Warry, 1998), and although Indigenous communities differ in their response to the trauma of marginalization and oppression, many Indigenous communities have been plagued by problems of family violence, substance abuse, incarceration and suicide (Canada, 2006a; Frank, 1992; Kirmayer, et al., 2003; Warry, 1998). The social and mental health problems that plague some communities are often interrelated and serve as indicators of larger family and community problems (Bohn, 2003; Frank, 1992). Issues of insufficient housing and infrastructure and poor access to recreational facilities are just a few examples of factors that contribute to the self-perpetuating cycle of collective trauma and destructive coping strategies through which community mental health problems persist (Canada, 2006a; Dion Stout & Kipling, 2003). Through intergenerational transmission of social burdens, mental health problems can become problems that are not only severe and persistent across an individual's lifetime, but also chronic across generations within a community. Given this knowledge, it should come as no surprise that healing approaches focused exclusively on individuals have demonstrated limited effectiveness among Aboriginal peoples (DeGagné, 2007; Mussell, et al., 2004). Healing strategies must consider the burden individual behaviours have had on family and community life (Warry, 1998). Thus, while individual healing is important for overall community healing, the strategies that will be most successful in achieving community wellness will promote both individual and collective healing (First Nations Centre, 2005; Warry, 1998).

8. The Impact of Chronic Diseases on Mental Health

The experiences of people with chronic diseases are an important aspect of the chronic disease research literature. An important sub-set of the experiences of chronic diseases is the impact that having a chronic disease has on one's mental health. Thus, the association between chronic disease and mental illness will be discussed in this section. In doing so, it will address three key questions: (1) how are chronic diseases and mental health related? (2) Why are chronic diseases and mental health related? And, (3) to what extent are chronic diseases and mental health related?

8.1 Defining the parameters of the association between chronic disease and mental health

The association between chronic disease and mental illness is often discussed as the interconnection between chronic disease and depression. As discussion in the "severe mental illness" section, it is often questioned whether depression is actually a chronic illness. "Major depression" is often the term used to refer to chronic depression. As noted, major depression has long-term effects on a patient's history, help-seeking behaviour, social environment, and on compliance to treatment (Van Weel-Baumgarten, 2005). Depressive symptoms below the threshold for major depression have been found to have significant effects on daily function, and health care utilization (Sullivan, et al., 1999) and are frequently precursors of more severe depression (Hammen, 1997). The prevalence of sub-threshold depressive symptoms is at least equal to that of major depression and may be as much as two to three times that of major depression (Sullivan, et al., 1999). As such, the interactions between chronic disease and all types of depression are important to examine. Following a discussion of depression, another psychological condition – adjustment disorder – that is related to the onset of chronic disease will be discussed.

8.1.1 Depression

The interconnection between chronic disease and depression is complex. Not only have some studies found that chronic diseases cause depression, but depression has been found to be independent risk factors for the development of certain types of chronic diseases. Depression is also associated with poorer outcomes, increased mortality and higher health care costs. The presence of depression influences health behaviours, making people less likely to make healthy lifestyle decisions or adhere to their medical treatment. Depression has been found to affect illness perceptions, making people who are depressed feel they are more ill than objective medical tests would predict. People who are depressed also have lower pain thresholds, making symptoms more painful than for an individual that was not depressed.

Depression can have direct physiological effects on disease such as in the case of diabetes, where depressive episodes have been associated with elevated glycemic levels. Among those with coronary heart disease, changes in lipid levels, physiological responses to stress and platelet function have all been explored for their relationship to depression (Davidson, et al., 2006; Glassman & Shapiro, 1998; Hippisley-Cox, Fielding, & Pringle, 1998; Lesperance, Frasure-Smith, & Talajic, 1996; Pratt, et al., 1996). In addition, some drugs used to treat chronic diseases have been known to cause depression (Katon & Sullivan, 1990) and some drugs used to treat depression have been shown to affect chronic disease, as in the case of older classes of antidepressants which have coronary effects (Davidson, et al., 2006; Pratt, et al., 1996). Depression can be a symptom of a chronic disease, as in the case of stroke (Fava & Kendler, 2000) and depressive symptoms can be confused with the signs and symptoms of heart disease.

8.1.2 Adjustment Disorder

Another psychological condition related to the onset of chronic disease is adjustment disorder. Most patients with chronic disease do not have clinical depressions but rather suffer from an 'adjustment disorder' which is stress-related, time limited, non-psychotic disturbance that initiates within three months post stressor onset and resolves within six months (Casey, 2001; O'Keeffe & Ranjith, 2007; Rush, Polatin, & Gatchel, 2000). Adjustment disorder is a serious condition that affects up to one quarter of patients of any age without any pre-existing mental disorder (Casey, 2001; Strain, et al., 1998) and complicates the course of medical conditions (Casey, 2001).

Adjustment disorders are seen as an understandable but maladaptive response to a stressful event that resolves spontaneously when the stressor is removed or a new level of adaptation is reached (O'Keeffe & Ranjith, 2007). Diagnosis is made when the criteria for more specific diagnosis such as depressive episode or major or minor depression are not met (Casey, 2001; Casey, et al., 2006; Takei & Sugihara, 2006). Some clinicians prefer to diagnose adjustment disorder rather than other depressive disorders because of their unwillingness to 'medicalize' what they feel is a natural reaction to illness (Casey, 2001; O'Keeffe & Ranjith, 2007); this is despite the fact that even the term adjustment disorder has been accused of pushing a human response to the realm of biomedicine.

Adjustment disorder encompasses serious mental symptoms and behaviours (Casey, 2001; Strain, et al., 1998) that are indistinguishable from other depression disorders on the basis of symptom severity (Casey, et al., 2006). Despite the fact that adjustment disorder shows similarly poor morbidity and mortality outcomes to those with other depressive disorders (Jones, Yates, Williams, Zhou, & Hardman, 1999; O'Keeffe & Ranjith, 2007), and that up to 15% of individuals go on to suffer a subsequent course of major depression (Takei & Sugihara, 2006), many clinicians are slow to provide treatment (Strain, et al., 1998). Casey (2001) explained this lack of treatment by suggesting that most individuals with adjustment disorder recover quickly and completely making it unlikely that specific interventions are required. For example, among those suffering from heart attacks, the risk of death has been associated with recurrent depression rather than a single episode of major depression occurring for the first time after a heart attack (Lesperance, Frasure-Smith, & Talajic, 1996). Depression is often more severe immediately following a myocardial infarction (MI) event and may be a transient reaction to the MI itself (Davidson, et al., 2006).

However, in the time immediately following the onset of the disease it is not possible to distinguish those who will recover over time and those who will go on to develop a major depressive disorder. Evidence suggests that patients with adjustment disorder can benefit from treatment as much as patients with other depressive disorders (Jones, et al., 1999) therefore treatment decisions must be balanced between the high prevalence of adjustment disorders, the significant time and resource required to treat them (Strain, et al., 1998) and the potential benefits to the patient. Perhaps because of its inherently short duration and relatively high recovery rates, very little research has been done on this condition (Casey, 2001; Casey, et al., 2006; O'Keeffe & Ranjith, 2007).

The distinction between the time-limited and disease-association of this disorder from major depression is critical to the rest of this chapter. The fact that so little research has been done on this disorder and the failure of adjustment disorders to be incorporated into recent studies may have resulted in the prevalence of depressive disorders in many research studies involving medical illness to be misrepresented. Casey et al. (2006) suggested that the number of mild depressive episodes and combined depressive episodes are being conflated in relation to the number of adjustment disorders.

Some authors have argued that the exact language in diagnosing patients is not relevant to the management of these patients (O'Keeffe & Ranjith, 2007). Rather than focusing on whether a patient has adjustment disorder, major or minor depression, O'Keeffe and Ranjith argue that a better approach would be to ask "what are the patient's current problems and how can we deal with them?". In this way, clinicians "would be able to use antidepressants for anhedonia, existential or spiritual approaches for demoralization, psycho-educational or cognitive approaches to deal with maladaptive adjustment and behavioural activation for poor motivation and learned helplessness, where indicated, in the same patient."

8.2 Unpacking the Associations between Chronic Disease and Mental Health

The challenge with defining and describing the association between chronic diseases in mental health is that there are many possible mechanisms for interactions between the two health conditions. The following table, which is an abbreviated version of one presented in Prince, Patel et al. (2007), exemplifies this.

Table 4. Possible mechanisms for interactions between mental disorders and other health conditions

Mental disorders affect the rate of other conditions

- Mental disorders are associated with risk factors for chronic disease such as smoking, reduced activity, poor diet, obesity, and hypertension; however, these lifestyle factors have not yet been shown to mediate associations with morbidity and mortality
- Depression has various biological effects: on serotonin metabolism (alteration of cardiac function, platelet aggregation, and vasoconstriction); on cortisol metabolism (increased cortisol, leading to inflammation, excessive clotting, and the metabolic syndrome); on inflammatory processes (raised inflammatory markers, which also predict the development of cardiovascular disease); and on cell-mediated immunity (impairments in T-cell mediated functions, reduced natural-killer cell counts and cytotoxicity, with relevance to cancer, HIV progression and other infectious disease)
- Mental disorders and other health conditions could have common genetic or environmental risk factors

Some health conditions affect the risk of mental disorders

- Many chronic diseases create a psychological burden, which arises from factors such as the acute trauma of the diagnosis; the difficulty of living with the illness; the long-term threat of decline and shortened life expectancy; necessary lifestyle changes; complicated therapeutic regimens; aversive symptoms such as pain; and stigma, which can lead to guilt, loss of social support, or breakdown of key relationships
- Disability associated with chronic health conditions might mediate risk for depression and other common mental disorders

Some co-morbid mental disorders affect treatment and outcome for other health conditions

- Mental disorders can delay help-seeking, reduce the likelihood of detection and diagnosis, or do both
- The extent and the quality of general medical health care received by people with mental disorders might be poor. This evidence for this inequity is especially strong for those with psychoses, dementia, and substance-use disorders
- Mental disorders, cognitive impairment, and substance use and alcohol-use disorders adversely affect adherence to medication, to recommendations for behavioural modification, and to activities to prevent disease or promote health.

Source: (Prince, et al., 2007).

The list of potential interactions is long, and recurring interactions between chronic physical disease and mental ill health are common, with each feeding into and exacerbating the other (Dowrick, 2006). Nevertheless, there is variability in prevalence of depression rates across different chronic diseases (Penninx, et al., 1996). Findings from this large body of research have been somewhat contradictory.

8.2.1 Variability in prevalence among chronic diseases

Some studies have found that there is little variability among chronic diseases in terms of psychological distress (Cassileth, et al., 1984). Others have shown that certain chronic diseases have elevated levels of psychological disturbance, including arthritis/rheumatism (Penninx, et al., 1996; Wells, Golding, & Burnam, 1988), cancer (Wells, et al., 1988), lung disease, neurological disorders, heart disease (Ormel, et al., 1997; Wells, et al., 1988), lower back pain (Carroll, Cassidy, & Coté, 2000; Rush, et al., 2000), stroke (Penninx, et al., 1996), hearing impairment, vision impairment (Ormel, et al., 1997), headache, and gastro-intestinal problems (Carroll, et al., 2000) and physical handicap. Finally, other studies have found that certain disorders are not associated with increased risk for psychological disturbance compared to other chronic conditions including hypertension (Patten, 1999; Wells, et al., 1988), arthritis (Patten, 1999), heart disease (Patten, 1999; Penninx, et al., 1996) and diabetes (Patten, 1999; Penninx, et al., 1996; Wells, et al., 1988). The fact that many of these conditions have been found to be both associated and not associated with increased psychological disturbance suggests that there is still much to learn about the relationship between depression and chronic disease.

Various reasons for the variation in psychological effect among different chronic diseases have been offered. It has been suggested that it is not the type of disease, but rather various other social and psychological factors that affects depression rates (Arpin, Fitch, Browne, & Corey, 1990). Some have suggested that the level of depression is directly associated to the severity of disability associated with the individual case of chronic disease (Ormel, et al., 1997). Others have suggested that the degree of manageability of the disease is most important. For example, unlike cancer or arthritis, diabetes and cardiac diseases are relatively manageable by individual or medical efforts, and modifying behaviour by changing diet, medication and physical exercise may improve their health. (Penninx, et al., 1996). Others have found that the meaning given to the illness is the most important factor influencing adjustment. Arpin, Fitch et al. found that the meaning given to illness, followed by family function, and disability variables accounted for 57% in the variance in adjustment outcomes (Arpin, et al., 1990).

8.2.2 Demographic variance

Among the non-Aboriginal population, major depression is most common among younger individuals and among women (Hammen, 1997). Depression is also more common among women in the Aboriginal population (H. V. Thommasen, et al., 2005; D. Wardman & Khan, 2004). Considering the young age of the Aboriginal population compared to the non-Aboriginal population, and the relatively young age at onset of chronic disease among Aboriginal peoples, the relationship between age, depression and chronic illness is of significance.

Cumulative epidemiological and clinically-based studies in the general literature have shown that children who have a chronic illness or disability are at a heightened risk for mental health problems (Cadman, Boyle, Szatmari, & Offord, 1987; Chernoff, Ireys, DeVet, & Kim, 2002; Haggerty, Roghmann, & Pless, 1975; Lavigne & Faier-Routman, 1992; R. E. Stein, Westbrook, & Silver, 1998; Suris, Michaud, & Viner, 2004; Wolman, Resnick, Harris, & Blum, 1994; Yeo & Sawyer, 2005). In addition, adolescents with chronic illness report higher emotional distress and suicidal tendencies than their counterparts and that they rank below their peers on a number of psychological outcomes including emotional well-being, worries and concerns, and body image (Miauton, Narring, & Michaud, 2003; Rosina, Crisp, & Steinbeck, 2003; Suris, et al., 2004; Wolman, et al., 1994).

Results from a population-based study revealed that the estimated prevalence of a psychiatric diagnosis among children with reported chronic illness was 10%, almost twice the rate found in children without chronic illness (Hysing, Elgen, Gillberg, Lie, & Lundervold, 2007). This is consistent with previous studies, the Isle of Wight study being the classic example, which found psychiatric disorders rates of between 11.6% among children with chronic physical disorders not involving the brain to 34.4% among children with neuro-epileptic conditions, compared to 7% of healthy children (Rutter, Graham, & Yule, 1970). A population-based study in Ontario in the 1980s found that children with both chronic illness and associated disability were at greater than threefold risk for psychiatric disorders and considerable risk for social adjustment problems. Children with chronic medical conditions, but no disability were at considerable less risk: about a twofold increase in psychiatric disorders but little increase risk for social adjustment problems was observed (Cadman, Boyle, Szatmari, & Offord, 1987).

Among First Nations adolescents, youth with disabilities seem more prone to depression, which is defined as feeling sad, blue or depressed for more than two weeks in a row in the reference year (35.6% compared to 26.5% of youth without disabilities). Adolescents with disabilities are also more likely to have contemplated committing suicide at some point in their lives (32.4% compared with 20.1%) (First Nations Centre, 2005).

8.2.3 Chronic diseases and mental health – the relationship within specific chronic conditions

In order to add to the discussion of the general variance in the relationship between chronic disease and mental health, literature documenting the particular relationship between three of the chronic diseases discussed earlier in this section: (1) diabetes, (2) cardiovascular disease and (3) musculoskeletal conditions. Information will be drawn from the general literature, with specific reference to the Aboriginal research when it is available.

Diabetes

In the Aboriginal population, diabetes research may arguably be the most prolific area of chronic disease research. Despite this, little research has addressed the mental health aspect of this disease. Perhaps this is because diabetes is also considered to be one of the most challenging chronic conditions from a psychosocial perspective (Gonder-Frederisk, Cox, & Clarke, 2002). This is because the diagnosis, treatment, and prevention is multifaceted and has a complex disease management structure:

> There is no cure, diagnosis can occur at any stage of life, and, after diagnosis, daily treatment is required for the remainder of the lifespan, which may or may not successfully prevent the development of serious long-term complications, such as cardiovascular and kidney disease. The management regimen can be enormously complex and relies almost solely on the intensive, daily efforts of patient and their families (Gonder-Frederisk, et al., 2002).

As a result, the interrelation between diabetes and mental health needs to be carefully unpacked. Research has begun to do this over the last thirty years; the outcomes of this work will be reviewed to describe the obviously complex relationships between diabetes and depression.

The relationship between diabetes and depression can be thought to go both ways: depression may play a role in the development and worsening of diabetes (Sacco, et al., 2007) or depression may be the result of living with a chronic condition and the ensuing decrease in quality of life (R. Anderson, Freedland, Clouse, & Lustman, 2001; Gonder-Frederisk, et al., 2002; Knol, et al., 2006; Peyrot & Rubin, 1997). Prospective studies have shown that people who have depression have up to double the risk of getting type 2 diabetes independent of other associated risk factors (Eaton, Armenian, Gallo, Pratt, & Ford, 1996; Kawakami, Takatsuka, Shimizu, & Ishibashi, 1999; Knol, et al., 2006). Retrospective studies have also found a greater propensity for a history of depression among diabetics than non-diabetics (R. Anderson, Lustman, Clouse, De Groot, & Freedland, 2000; Gonder-Frederisk, et al., 2002; Lustman, Griffith, Freedland, Kissel, & Clouse, 1998; Nichols & Brown, 2000; Peyrot & Rubin, 1997). Exact estimates range, but generally individuals with diabetes suffer depression at rates of two to three times that of the general population – affecting as many as one-third of individuals with type 1 or type 2 diabetes (R. Anderson, et al., 2001; R. Anderson, et al., 2000; Gonder-Frederisk, et al., 2002).

Depression in diabetes is associated with higher blood glucose levels, poor glycemic control, poorer lifestyle and medication adherence, decreased quality of life, substantially higher health care costs, increased risk for complications and increased mortality (R. Anderson, et al., 2001; Egede, 2005; Gavard, Lustman, & Clouse, 1993; Goldney, Phillips, Fisher, & Wilson, 2004; Gonder-Frederisk, et al., 2002; Kawakami, et al., 1999; McGill, et al., 1992; Peyrot & Rubin, 1997; Sacco, et al., 2007; Winokur, Maislin, Phillips, & Amsterdam, 1988). Depressed diabetic patients have been shown to have elevated blood sugar levels during a depressive episode and longer recovery times than non-depressed subjects (Winokur, Maislin, Phillips, & Amsterdam, 1988). Often depression can be a stronger predictor of disease outcomes than physiological variables (Knol, et al., 2006; Rubin & Peyrot, 1999). Chronic anxiety has been shown to be related to glycosylated haemoglobin HbA1c, a measure of diabetic control. The same study found that improvements in anxiety might be useful in controlling glucose metabolism (Okada, et al., 1995).

In Canada, only one study was found that provided insight into the relationship between quality of life, diabetes and depression among Aboriginal peoples. This study found that Aboriginal people have lower quality of life than non-Aboriginal people and that the average number of unhealthy days for mental health was higher among Aboriginal than for non-Aboriginal people (H. V. Thommasen, et al., 2005). Only a few studies conducted in the United States of America have examined the prevalence of depressive symptoms among Indigenous peoples with diabetes (Bell, et al., 2005; Sahmoun, Markland, & Helgerson, 2007; Singh, et al., 2004; Tann, Yabiku, Okamoto, & Yanow, 2007). These studies have found inconsistent results. Some studies showed rates of depressive symptoms several times more prevalent among Native Americans with diabetes than among other ethnicities (Tann, Yabiku, Okamoto, & Yanow, 2007), other Native American non-diabetics (Sahmoun, Markland, & Helgerson, 2007; Singh, et al., 2004), and greater, but not significantly so, than other ethnic minorities (Bell, et al., 2005). Other studies found no association between race and measures of depression when other demographic and disease factors were controlled (Peyrot & Rubin, 1997). The dearth of studies on ethnic minorities, and Aboriginal peoples in particular, means that little is known about the prevalence of depression among the Aboriginal diabetic population, regional variations, demographic and medical characteristics associated with higher depression, medical outcomes associated with depression, health care utilization, or effective and culturally-appropriate treatments (Bell, et al., 2005; Rock, 2003).

The literature has documented a relationship between depression and diabetic complications (de Groot, Anderson, Freedland, Clouse, & Lustman, 2001): although the direction of the relationship is not clear. Diabetics who are depressed are at increased risk for diabetes-related complications and the greater the number or severity of diabetic complications the higher the level of depression (de Groot, Anderson, Freedland, Clouse, & Lustman, 2000; de Groot, et al., 2001; Peyrot & Rubin, 1997). Depression may play a part in some complications (e.g. macrovascular disease) but not on other complications (e.g. nephropathy) (de Groot, et al., 2001). Since certain types of complications are more prevalent among Aboriginal peoples (e.g. renal complications (A. Hanley, et al., 2005) and that Aboriginal peoples have higher rates of diabetes complications than among the non-Aboriginal population (A. Hanley, et al., 2005; Meatherall, et al., 2005;

Simpson, Corabian, Jacobs, & Johnson, 2003), a better understanding of the relationship between depression and the complications most common for Aboriginal people, nephropathy for example, is needed.

Cardiovascular Disease

As noted earlier, cardiovascular disease (CVD) is a heterogeneous group of diseases of the heart and blood vessels, of which coronary heart disease or ischemic heart disease is the most common. While CVD has been found to be slightly higher in the First Nations population, rates among other Aboriginal groups are limited. When discussing CVD it is important to note its interrelation with diabetes and diabetes risk factors (S. G. Bruce, et al., 2003; Simpson, Corabian, Jacobs, & Johnson, 2003). This is important in the Aboriginal context, as diabetes and CVD have both been found to have high prevalence rates. Further, diabetics who suffer from depression are at an increased risk for cardiovascular disease: depression has been found to be an independent risk factor for the development of coronary heart disease among those with diabetes (R. Anderson, Freedland, Clouse, & Lustman, 2001). Egede (2005) found that those with for diabetes and depression were at significantly greater risk for death from all causes beyond that due to having either diabetes or depression alone, although diabetes remained a stronger predictor of coronary heart disease mortality than depression. The research on the interrelation between CVD and depression will be reviewed in greater detail below.

Cross-sectional and case-control studies have shown that rates of depression are higher among patients with coronary-artery disease than among the general population (Pratt, et al., 1996). Up to 20% of patients with heart disease meet the criteria for major depression (Davidson, et al., 2006), three times the community-based prevalence (Rozanski, Blumenthal, & Kaplan, 1999). Between 15-45% of patients admitted to hospital following myocardial infarction (MI) are depressed and 40-50% report moderate to severe levels of anxiety (P. Bennett & Carroll, 1997; Glassman & Shapiro, 1998; Hippisley-Cox, Fielding, & Pringle, 1998).

Depression has been deemed to be an independent risk factor on par with other known medical prognostic factors as a risk factor for the development and the worsening of cardiovascular disease (Broadley, Korszun, Jones, & Frenneaux, 2002; Davidson, et al., 2006; Frasure-Smith & Lesperance, 2005; Glassman & Shapiro, 1998; Hippisley-Cox, Fielding, & Pringle, 1998;

T. Smith & Ruiz, 2002; Sullivan, et al., 1999). A number of studies support the notion of a gradient between the magnitude of depression and future cardiac events, suggesting that risk for coronary artery disease associated with depression exists along a continuum, with the relative risk depending on the magnitude of depressive symptoms (Glassman & Shapiro, 1998; Rozanski, et al., 1999).

Among patients with pre-existing cardiovascular disease, depression has consistently been associated with a worse outcome (Carver, 2007; Glassman & Shapiro, 1998). Estimates of the effects of depression on heart disease vary from study to study but range from a one-and-a-half- to seven-fold risk of fatal cardiac events (Broadley, et al., 2002; Davidson, et al., 2006; Frasure-Smith & Lesperance, 2000; Pratt, et al., 1996). Depression is also associated with adverse medical outcomes such as poor compliance, increased health care utilization (Gilmer, et al., 2005), increased morbidity and mortality, and decreased quality of life (Davidson, et al., 2006; Hippisley-Cox, et al., 1998; Lustman, Griffith, Freedland, & Clouse, 1997), even at low levels (Davidson, et al., 2006). One study found an increased risk for cardiac mortality or MI among 72% of its participants reporting only two symptoms of depression, a level of depression insufficient to diagnose major or even minor depression (Horsten, Mittleman, Wamala, Schenck-Gustafsson, & Orth-Gomér, 2000). Among those who have suffered a heart attack higher levels of depression or anxiety is associated with increased mortality and morbidity, poor emotional recovery, lack of short term improvement, and longer latency to normal levels of activity (P. Bennett & Carroll, 1997; Gorkin, Follick, Wilkin, & Niaura, 1994; Pratt, et al., 1996; T. Smith & Ruiz, 2002).

A study among Australia Aborigine people found that stress and worry relating to the changing social situation within the community were frequently identified as a perceived cause of heart disease and as a complicating factor in managing it. The community saw heart disease as a symbol of contemporary social problems and of uncertain community direction (Ong & Weeramanthri, 2002). Citing Humphrey et al. 1998, Ong and Weeramanthri (2002) state that the stress and worry experienced by Indigenous people was often not recognized as such by non-Indigenous people, who see stress as being solely related to a modern lifestyle and overwork. As Skinner and Silverman-Peach (1989) describes, non-Indian health care providers often misperceive the stoic demeanour of Indian people (in the presence of non-Indians) as indicating the absence of stress (Skinner & Silverman-Peach, 1989).

Musculoskeletal Diseases

As noted in the musculoskeletal burden section, arthritis is one of the most prevalent chronic health conditions in Canada and a major cause of morbidity, disability and health care utilization (Lagacé, Perruccio, DesMeules, & Badley, 2003). Much of the literature reports on the prevalence of musculoskeletal conditions using the heading 'arthritis/rheumatism' to refer to this collection of painful joint disorders that range from those related to wear and tear of cartilage (osteoarthritis) to those associated with inflammation resulting from an immune disorder (rheumatoid arthritis). As such, it is often too difficult to separate these two conditions. While the relation between arthritis and osteoarthritis, and mental health will be referred to wherever possible information, statistics related to arthritis/rheumatism will also be used.

Rates of arthritis/rheumatism are 1.5 times higher among First Nations/Inuit than among the general Canadian population (First Nations Centre, 2004) As such, among Aboriginal adults, arthritis/rheumatism is the most commonly reported chronic condition (Health Canada, 2003a) with an age standardized prevalence of 27% compared to 16% among the non-Aboriginal population (First Nations Centre, 2005; Lagacé, et al., 2003). Since the prevalence of arthritis/rheumatism increases with age (Lagacé, et al., 2003) the impact of arthritis/rheumatism on the Aboriginal population is expected to increase as the population continues to age (Burke, Zautra, Schultz, Reich, & Davis, 2002).

Figure 5. Proportion of individuals with arthritis who reported an HUI score indicative of disability, by age, Aboriginal people living off reserve and non-Aboriginal people, household population aged 15 years and over, Canada, 2000

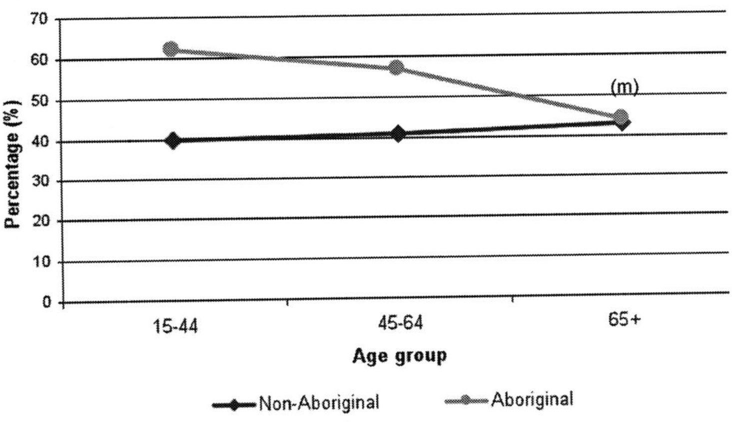

Source: (Lagacé, et al., 2003).

Note: Differences between Aboriginals living off-reserve and non-Aboriginals are statistically significant at $p < 0.05$ except for people aged 65 years and over. (m) indicates that the coefficient of variation is between 16.6% and 33.3%.

Individuals with arthritis are more likely than people with other chronic conditions and no chronic conditions to suffer from activity limitations, increased disability, and moderate to severe pain (Lagacé, et al., 2003; Verbrugge, Lepkowski, & Konkol, 1991). Verbrugge, Lepowski et al. (1991) found that comparing arthritic and non-arthritic people with the same total number of conditions, arthritis people had more physical limitations of all kinds (Verbrugge, et al., 1991). They also found that when arthritis co-occurs with other chronic conditions, disability levels are augmented considerably. For example, for walking, Verbrugge, Lepowski et al. (1991) found that there was an over one hundred-fold increase in disability risk for people with both arthritis and other chronic conditions (odds ratio 113.3) compared to an odds ration of 46.5 for the people with other (non arthritis) chronic conditions. Aboriginal people with arthritis also have been found to have higher rates of disability than non-Aboriginals with arthritis, as exemplified in Figure 5 (Lagacé, et al., 2003).

As disability and pain are all associated with increased risk of depression, those with arthritis/rheumatism are at particular risk of depression (Barlow, Cullen, & Rowe, 1999). Individuals with arthritis/rheumatism experience more depression than the general population (Barlow, et al., 1999; Dickens, McGowan, Clark-Carter, & Creed, 2002; Hawley & Wolfe, 1993; Lagacé, et al., 2003; Lin, et al., 2003; Nagyoca, Stewart, Macejova, van Dijk, & van de Heuval, 2005; Nicassio, 2008; Treharne, Kitas, Lyons, & Booth, 2005) with depression rates between 17% and 42% being reported (Ang, Choi, Kroenke, & Wolfe, 2005; Evers, Kraaimaat, Geenen, & Bijlsma, 1997; R. Frank, et al., 1988; Hawley & Wolfe, 1993; Rosemann, et al., 2007) though not higher than those with other chronic conditions (Newman, 1997). Out of patients with moderately severe to severe symptoms of depression, only 19% discussed depression during their medical visits, and patients had to initiate the discussion with their provider each time (Sleath, et al., 2008).

Figure 6. Proportion of individuals with case depression, by age, Canada, 2000

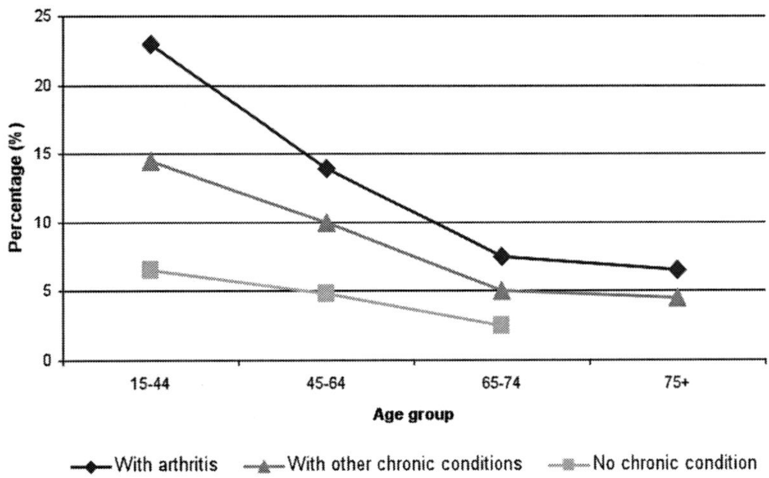

Source: (Lagacé, et al., 2003).

Note: Values for people with arthritis are significantly higher than values for people with other and no chronic conditions at $p < 0.05$. Because of the small sample size, data for people aged 75+ years in the "no chronic condition" group cannot be released.

The relationship between rheumatoid arthritis and depression has received more attention in the literature than the relationship between osteoarthritis and depression (Wolfe, 1999). Some studies have found that those with rheumatoid arthritis are more depressed than those with osteoarthritis (Dickens, McGowan, Clark-Carter, & Creed, 2002). Other studies however have not found depressive scores to be higher or more common among patients with rheumatoid arthritis (Hawley & Wolfe, 1993). Given that most First Nations individuals with arthritis suffer from osteoarthritis[10] (First Nations and Inuit Regional Health Survey National Steering Committee, 1999) the majority of the research available is not on the condition most prevalent among Aboriginal peoples. While rheumatoid arthritis is not the focus of our interest in chronic musculoskeletal conditions, the research that has been done in this area may be beneficial to better understanding the association between arthritis, osteoarthritis, and depression in Aboriginal communities.

10 Surveys such as the FNIRHS do ask about "arthritis and rheumatism" but cannot distinguish the various diagnostic varieties. Most respondents who report having arthritis most likely suffer from osteoarthritis (First Nations and Inuit Regional Health Survey National Steering Committee, 1999)

Some authors, for example, have found that the time since onset of illness is important. Treharne, Kitas et al. (1995) found that those with established rheumatoid arthritis were significantly less depressed than those recently diagnosed. Others have found no difference in depression between recently diagnosed and chronic patients in terms of the distress they experience (Barlow, et al., 1999; Barlow, Cullen, & Rowe, 2002; Evers, et al., 1997). One study found that the strongest predictors of depression severity were perceived pain, few social contacts, physical limitation of the lower body and upper body, age, and body mass index (Rosemann, et al., 2007). Another found that sex, pain and functional status, disease-related impact on daily life, and perceived social support were related to psychological distress among those recently diagnosed (Evers, Kraaimaat, Geenen, & Bijlsma, 1997). Another study, on the other hand, did not find that pain was a significant predictor of depressive symptoms. Rather, beliefs about accepting one's illness and fatigue were more influential (Barlow, et al., 1999).

Unlike other chronic illnesses there does not appear to be any suggestion of depression playing an etiological role in the onset of arthritis/rheumatism (Rosemann, et al., 2007). Rather depression is seen as an additional burden that affects adjustment to the condition and ultimately the disease outcome (Burke, et al., 2002). Comorbid depression in individuals with arthritis has been shown to be an independent predictor of all-cause mortality with patients with persistent or recurrent depression twice more likely to die than patients with no depression (Ang, Choi, Kroenke, & Wolfe, 2005).

A direct relationship between the physical markers of the extent or activity of the disease and depression has not been found (Newman, 1997). Research has shown that objective physiological measures of disease are not as robust a predictor of disability as psychological factors such as depression and pain (Botha-Scheepers, et al., 2006; Kee, 2003; Lin, et al., 2003).

8.3 Common themes

As is certainly evident from the above discussion, there are some themes common to chronic diseases that have a potential impact on one's mental health and can predispose individuals with chronic diseases to depression. The common themes of disability, quality of life, illness perception, self-perceptions, and self-control will be discussed briefly below.

8.3.1 Level of Disability

The relationship between level of disability and depression extends across many chronic conditions and has been explored within the context of the different conditions. The prevalence of chronic conditions has been associated with activity limitation among First Nations and Inuit populations in Canada, with 24% of people with hypertension, 28% of those with diabetes, 33% of those with arthritis, 36% of those with heart disease, and 38% of those with cancer reporting some degree of activity limitation (First Nations Centre, 2004). It has been found that those with increased disability suffer from poorer mental health (Barlow, et al., 1999; Cadman, et al., 1987; Cassileth, et al., 1984; Covington, 1991) and those with poor mental health have increased disability (Patten, 1999; Penninx, Leveille, Ferrucci, van Eijk, & Guralnik, 1999; Scott, et al., 2008; Sullivan, et al., 1999).

A population-based study in Ontario in the 1980s found that children with both chronic illness and associated disability were at a greater than threefold risk for psychiatric disorders while children with only chronic medical conditions but no disability had only a twofold increase (Cadman, et al., 1987). Penninx, Beekman et al. (1996) found that diseases involving more functional impairments such as stroke and arthritis had relatively stronger associations with psychological distress than other chronic diseases that had less functional limitations such as diabetes, cardiac disease and cancer. In contrast, some studies have found that among individuals living with chronic illness, decreases in physical functioning and advancement of chronic conditions were not associated with equal decreases in mental health, perhaps due to a process of psychological adaptation (Singer, Hopman, & MacKenzie, 1999). Overall, the research has shown that Aboriginal peoples suffer greater disability than the general Canadian population. Among First Nations adults with diabetes, roughly one-quarter experience activity limitations due to the disease (First Nations Centre, 2005). Figure 7 presents data on the activity limitations of First Nations living with diabetes as reported in the 1997 First Nations and Inuit Regional Health Survey.

Figure 7. Prevalence of disability among First Nations people with diabetes, percentage rates

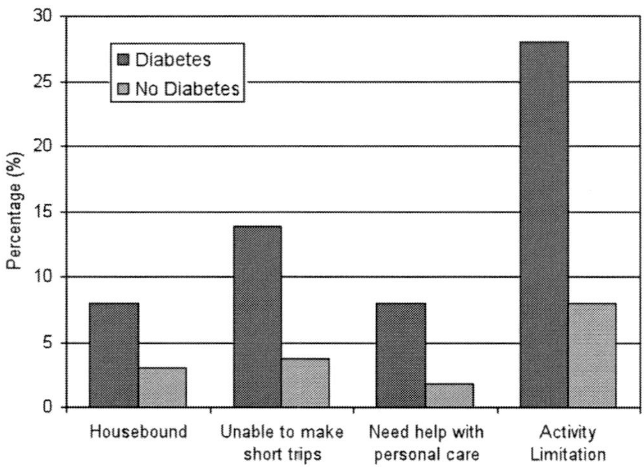

Source: (First Nations and Inuit Regional Health Survey National Steering Committee, 1999).

Mental health disorders have also been shown to have negative effects on disability, at a rate equal to that of common chronic physical conditions (Schonfeld, et al., 1997; Scott, et al., 2008). One study found that depression in initially non-disabled older adults with chronic conditions significantly increased the risk for disability, especially for arthritis and angina (Penninx, Leveille, Ferrucci, van Eijk, & Guralnik, 1999). In a study by Scott, Von Korff et al. (2008), individuals with mental disorder were more likely to be severely disabled than those with the physical conditions they investigated (diabetes, respiratory disease, headache, heart disease, arthritis, back or neck pain). They also found a synergistic effect between mental health and physical conditions: those with both mental and physical conditions were more likely to be severely disabled than those with either condition alone and had a greater likelihood than the sum of the odds of each condition individually. Directly related to disability is the impact of the association between chronic disease and mental health and quality of life. This is discussed below.

8.3.2 Impact on Quality of Life

Health-related quality of life refers to the ways in which health, illness, and medical treatment influence an individual's perception of functioning and well-being. Depression, chronic diseases, and quality of life are closely related although the direction of the relationship is not clear (Jacobson, de Groot, & Samson, 1997). Studies done with regards to people with diabetes found that diabetics with a diagnosis of depression have significantly lower quality of life compared with diabetics who are not depressed (Goldney, Phillips, Fisher, & Wilson, 2004; Gonder-Frederisk, et al., 2002; Jacobson, et al., 1994; H. Thommasen, Berkowitz, Thommasen, & Michalos, 2005). The effect of depression on quality of life was found to be greater than the effect of diabetes on quality of life (Goldney, et al., 2004). When just considering the impact of diabetes on quality of life, it was found that individuals with diabetes have considerably worse quality of life compared to the general population (Gonder-Frederisk, et al., 2002; Jacobson, et al., 1997; Mayou, Bryant, & Turner, 1990; Rubin & Peyrot, 1999; Steed, Cooke, & Newman, 2003). The reason for this is likely multifactoral. People with diabetes tend to be overweight, engage in less physical activity and are more likely to have medical co-morbidities (Gonder-Frederisk, et al., 2002; Jacobson, et al., 1997; H. Thommasen, et al., 2005). Better quality of life is associated with low blood glucose levels and tight metabolic control (Jacobson, et al., 1997; Rubin & Peyrot, 1999). In Canada, only one study was found that provided insight into the relationship between quality of life, diabetes and depression among Aboriginal peoples. This study found that Aboriginal people have lower quality of life than non-Aboriginal people and that the average number of unhealthy days for mental health was higher among Aboriginal people than for non-Aboriginal people (H. Thommasen, et al., 2005). As the majority of information in this area has focused on diabetes, research on the impact of other chronic diseases and their association with mental health on quality of life will be important to engage with in the future.

8.3.3 Illness perceptions and self-perceived health status

Illness perceptions and illness acceptance influence depression in individuals living with chronic diseases (Stanton & Revenson, 2007). Illness perceptions are the beliefs that patients hold about their illness, its effects, why it has happened, how long it will last and whether it can be cured or controlled (Botha-Scheepers, et al., 2006). Among those with arthritis/rheumatism, illness perceptions have been shown to have a strong impact on outcomes (Botha-Scheepers, et al., 2006). For example, a patient who sees the illness as negative, uncontrollable, and chronic are more likely to adjust poorly to the illness, report greater disability, have lower life satisfaction and suffer from greater depression, anxiety, pain, and fatigue (Botha-Scheepers, et al., 2006; Kee, 2003; Nagyoca, Stewart, Macejova, van Dijk, & van de Heuval, 2005; Treharne, Kitas, Lyons, & Booth, 2005). Alternatively, a person who accepts their chronic disease is able to set up new reasonable frames or goals and be able to fulfill them (Nagyoca, et al., 2005). Arpin, Fitch et al. (1990) found that the meaning given to illness was the largest contributor to the variance in adjustment outcomes observed among individuals with chronic illnesses, regardless of the type of illness or its severity. They then suggested that since there is no relationship between the severity of disease and the meaning given to the illness, unfavourable attitudes towards illness should be used to identify subjects in need of psychosocial services (Arpin, et al., 1990).

Research among American Indians with rheumatoid and osteoarthritis found that individuals expected to have decreased functional abilities and increasing pain and suffering (Kramer, Harker, & Wong, 2002). The same research found that negative thoughts, which have been associated with poor psychological outcomes and greater physical disability were generally absent (Kramer, et al., 2002). McCubbin, Thompson et al. (1993) found that Native American Indians defined the meaning of disability as part of a more general pattern of harmony disharmony, and viewed individuals with chronic conditions as a valued, functioning member of society rather than as some one that is different or stigmatized.

Self-perceived health status has also been found to be an important factor affecting depression among those with chronic disease. Among First Nations, self-perceived health has been related to suicide, the most dramatic indicators of distress. Suicidal thoughts were found to be more common among those with fair or poor rated health (38.4%) than among those with excellent self-reported health (28.9%) (First Nations Centre, 2005). Figure 8 illustrates self-perceived health status of First Nations living on reserve and other adults in Canada as reported in the 2002/03 RHS.

Figure 8. Self reported general health of First Nations and other adults in Canada

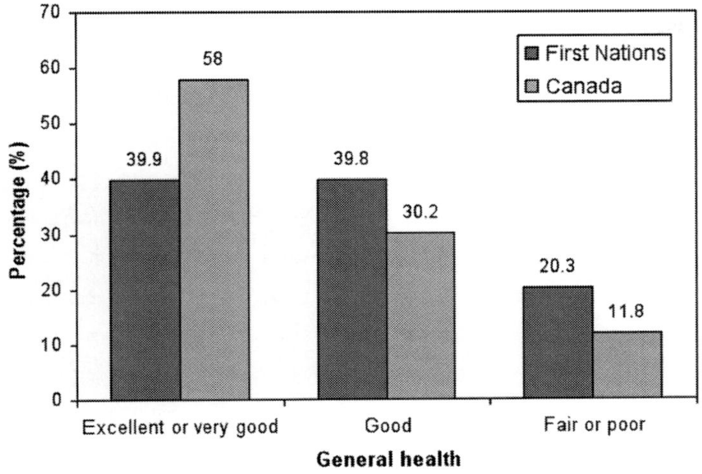

Source: (First Nations Centre, 2005).

Optimism is associated with less anxiety, depression and more life satisfaction among individuals suffering from rheumatoid arthritis. There is also evidence that people with a sense of high self-esteem, control and optimism adjust more successfully to chronic illness (Helgeson & Reynolds, 2002). Optimism has been associated with lower pain at initial onset of arthritis and interestingly higher pain for those with established disease, reflecting possibly unmet expectations of improvement or betterment of their condition (Treharne, et al., 2005).

8.3.4 Body Image and Self-esteem

In a similar way to one's perception of disease, self-esteem has been found to be associated with both physical and psychological health. While no research directly examines the relationship between self-esteem, depression and chronic disease among Aboriginal peoples, studies in other populations and with regards to one or more of these areas can be used to begin to unpack the relationship. For example, low self-esteem has been found to double the risk for later depression. Among individuals with rheumatoid arthritis, higher levels of self esteem, along with better adjustment to the illness were associated with less psychological distress (Nagyoca, et al., 2005). Body image and self-esteem have been particularly linked to the psychological health among those with chronic illnesses among adolescents.

A study by Wolman et al. (1994) found that body image was the most important predictor of emotional well-being for students with chronic conditions, suggesting that a strong sense of self (i.e. body image) as well as family cohesion and support were more important than having a disability on positive emotional development. Adolescents in British Columbia with chronic illnesses or disabilities are more likely than those without to have low self-esteem (17% vs. 5% respectively) (The McCreary Centre Society, 1994). Among First Nations youth with disabilities, 78.2% are somewhat less likely to agree or strongly agree with the statement "I like the way I am" compared to 85.6% among youth without disabilities. The difference is most pronounced among males, among whom 79.6% with disabilities agree or strongly agree with the statement compared to 90.4% of their counterparts without disabilities (First Nations Centre, 2005). In addition to a sense of comfort and pride in one's body and personal ability, sense of control over one's lives is also interconnected with chronic diseases and mental health.

8.3.5 Mastery

A sense of mastery refers to the extent to which people see themselves as in control of their lives (De Marco, 2000). Low perceived mastery includes feelings of helplessness and is associated with worse health and psychological outcomes (M. Daniel, O'Dea, Rowley, McDermott, & Kelly, 1999; Gonder-Frederisk, et al., 2002). Lower feelings of mastery may be more frequent among those with chronic illnesses because of the progressive physical deterioration and unpredictable symptom flare-ups common in many chronic diseases (Helgeson & Reynolds, 2002), and the greater likelihood of individuals with chronic illness or physical disability to be confronted with problems that are not amenable to problem solving (Penninx, et al., 1996). A high sense of mastery has been linked to improved physical and psychological health status among individuals with arthritis (Barlow, Cullen, & Rowe, 2002; Burke, et al., 2002) and among Aboriginal peoples, good mastery skills have been associated with healthy blood lipid levels (Mark Daniel, Rowley, Herbert, O'Dea, & Green, 2001) and low fasting glucose levels (Mark Daniel, Gamble, Henderson, & Burgess, 1995). Similarly, American research has found an inverse relationship between arthritis pain among American Indians and a sense of mastery (Kramer, et al., 2002). Another study found that individuals with arthritis and very high self-efficacy had higher pain thresholds and higher pain tolerance, while those with low self-efficacy had greater physical impairment, more pain, more fatigue, more depression and anxiety and less acceptance of their condition (Barlow, et al., 2002). One study among women with physical disabilities found that women equipped with high levels of personal resources (sense of mastery, self-esteem, or hardiness) had significantly better long-term psychosocial adaptation: perhaps due to their ability to better cope with the daily hardships and familial role difficulties of their illness and to use their limited concrete resources more efficiently (Dangoor & Florian, 1994).

The 2002/03 RHS asked questions closely relating to mastery, and the results (see Table 5 below) differ among those who were and were not depressed. Among adult First Nations who were depressed, only 28% strongly believed that they had control over things that happened to them, 7.4% felt helpless in dealing with problems of life and 10.6% strongly believed that there was little they could do to change many of the important things in their lives. The RHS found a similar pattern among youth with disability (First Nations Centre, 2005).

Table 5. Self-determination indicators by feelings of depression or sadness

% Strongly agreeing that...	Depressed	
	Yes	No
I can solve the problems I have	32.4%	38.5%
No one pushes me around in life	33.8%	41.0%
I have control over things that happen to me	28.0%	31.1% (NS)
I can do just about anything I set my mind to	35.2%	43.2%
I often feel helpless in dealing with the problems of life	7.4%	4.1%
What happens to me in the future mostly depends on me	37.0%	37.6% (NS)
There's little I can do to change many of the important things in my life	10.6%	5.9%

Source: (First Nations Centre, 2005).

Unfortunately, feelings of powerlessness and a low degree of controllability over the elements that affect their lives are common in many Aboriginal communities, largely as a result of the ongoing impacts of colonization (Boston, et al., 1997; Grams, et al., 1996). This powerlessness has long been recognized as a major factor shaping Aboriginal health (Tsey & Every, 2000).

Part IV: Conclusion

Health is determined by factors that include a plethora of inter-related domains including economic, social, political, spiritual and cultural. That Aboriginal peoples in Canada and Indigenous peoples abroad have been dislocated from their traditional ways of living and often excluded from full participation in the dominant settler societies, is understood.

Words are very important because they situate the Aboriginal health discourse in a space that recognizes a multi-dimensionality to the lived experience. Historically, social exclusion leads to economic marginalization which in turn creates inequality of opportunity, leading to greater risk and health disparities (described in this book) which finally renders communities vulnerable to disease, disability and death.

This book was intended to frame health in the broader social context. To highlight many population health indicators where a profound difference is evident when Aboriginal peoples are compared to their non-Aboriginal counterparts, to promote a life course approach to aboriginal health and to focus on the opportunity for community level intervention to create and evaluate programs addressing the factors which could optimize developmental trajectories to improve aboriginal population health and community well being.

In the process of illuminating profound disparities between Aboriginal People and the Canadian mainstream, the book contributes to a long tradition in Canadian Public Health, that being the construction of negative images about what the world thinks about being aboriginal in Canada. There is a problem in population and public health research which is referred to as 'epidemiologic bias' where, in the context of aboriginal health, studies about healthy aboriginal people and communities are, with rare exceptions, not accepted for publication because they do not conform to the preconceived notions held by reviewers and editors; that aboriginal health is all about aboriginal people being unhealthy.

The widespread feeling in Aboriginal communities is that of being 'Researched to Death' which means, in part, that research consistently depicts Aboriginal Peoples in negative ways, creating the illusion that all Aboriginal People are unhealthy and reinforcing unequal power relations which serve to support the status quo - that, Aboriginal peoples are not ready to manage their own affairs. Ironically, self determination has been recognized as the path forward toward improved health.

The truth is that while statistics paint a grim picture and need to be used to target public health efforts, not all aboriginal people are unhealthy. In fact, many communities are healthier on average than non-native people. How can this be when statistics point to profound disparity? The answer is that not all Aboriginal communities are the same. In fact, quite the opposite is the case. Extreme poverty and ill health are concentrated in some aboriginal communities but not all. So the question is fundamental to population health: why are some aboriginal communities healthy and other not? I don't know the answers but I do know that they need to come from communities, not imposed by well meaning government or outsiders.

First Nation, Inuit and Metis communities are making improvements in critical areas of education, employment, economic development and there is a renaissance of tradition and pride. The problem with Public and Population Health reporting is that it is historically driven by the medical model; often about ill health, dysfunction, disability and untimely death. Transformative research needs to improve health, minimize negative stereotyping and stigma, it needs to focus on what can be done to promote health informed by appropriate community interventions that leave something of benefit to the communities after the process of doing the research has been completed.

The health of populations is also determined by timely access to health services including medical and surgical intervention, preventative measures, rehabilitation services, transportation to health facilities, integrated primary care and public health. Community infrastructure, adequate housing and home care, personal security and living a life that is free of discrimination and racism are also factors related to optimizing health and well being.

There is no panacea but change is happening, led by interventions that are well conceived and well received. The narrowing of the gap in health is a complex and multi-faceted goal that will require attention to a broad variety of pre-disposing factors and a whole of government approach toward multi-sectored interventions.

Communities need to be true partners with researchers, government and other sponsors if practices that hold promise for sustainable economic development are to be successful. It is the communities that should be setting their own priorities and creating the yardstick by which success will be measured.

Clearly, a need exists to improve health and education to promote access to employment and income. Fundamentally, the eradication of poverty is a necessary precursor for improved health because many of the other health determinants, like adequate food and shelter, need to be purchased.

In summary, this book has attempted to look at old problems in an innovative way. The life course perspective is integrated as a connected whole and the goal is to improve population health determinants through healthy public policy while creating opportunities for improved health by clearly targeting specific life stages and gender issues to optimize healthy growth and development.

Finally, this book is a starting point for research. Readers are encouraged to go to both the academic published and unpublished 'grey' literature to obtain the most up to date information available and to use the latest evidence to inform new programs, policy and investigation.

Only by examining the current burden of chronic diseases borne by Aboriginal peoples and the risk factors associated with these diseases across the life course, and creating interventions to address health concerns; can future plans for action be established to begin to improve health and well being for Aboriginal peoples and in the process improve the health of all Canadians.

Works Cited

Adelson, N. (2005). The embodiment of inequity: health disparities in aboriginal Canada. *Can J Public Health, 96 Suppl 2*, S45-61.

Anand, S. S., Yusuf, S., Jacobs, R., Davis, A. D., Yi, Q. L., Gerstein, H., et al. (2001). Risk factors, atherosclerosis, and cardiovascular disease among Aboriginal people in Canada: the Study of Health Assessment and Risk Evaluation in Aboriginal Peoples (SHARE-AP). *Lancet, 358*(9288), 1147-1153.

Andersen, P., & Doherty, T. M. (2005). The success and failure of BCG-implications for a novel tuberculosis vaccine. *Nat Rev Microbiol, 3*(8), 656-662.

Anderson, H. R. (1978). Respiratory abnormalities in Papua New Guinea children: the effects of locality and domestic wood smoke pollution. *Int J Epidemiol, 7*(1), 63-72.

Anderson, J. (2003). Aboriginal Children in Poverty in Urban Communities: Social exclusion and the growing racialization of poverty in Canada, from http://www.ccsd.ca/pr/2003/aboriginal.htm

Anderson, R., Freedland, K., Clouse, R., & Lustman, P. (2001). The prevalence of cormorbid depression in adults with diabetes: A meta-analysis. *Diabetes Care, 24*(6), 1069-1078.

Ang, D. C., Choi, H., Kroenke, K., & Wolfe, F. (2005). Comorbid depression is an independent risk factor for mortality in patients with rheumatoid arthritis. *The Journal of Rheumatology, 32*, 1013-1019.

Arpin, K., Fitch, M., Browne, G., & Corey, P. (1990). Prevalence and correlates of family dysfunction and poor adjustment to chronic illness in specialty clinics *Journal of Clinical Epidemiology, 43*(4), 373-383.

Australia. Department of Employment Education and Training (1990). *Aboriginal Student Support and Parent Awareness (Asspa) Program: 1990 National Program Guidelines*. Australia: Commonwealth Government.

Bachrach, L. L. (1988). Defining Chronic Mental Illness: A Concept Paper. *Hospital and Community Psychiatry, 39*(4), 383-388.

Barker, D. J. (1995a). The fetal and infant origins of disease. *Eur J Clin Invest., 25*(7), 457.

Barker, D. J. (1995b). Fetal origins of coronary heart disease. *BMJ (Clinical research ed.), 311*(6998), 171.

Barker, D. J. (1995c). Intrauterine programming of adult disease. *Mol Med Today, 1*(9), 418-423.

Barker, D. J. (2004). Developmental origins of adult health and disease. *J Epidemiol Community Health, 58*(2), 114-115.

Barlow, J., Cullen, L., & Rowe, I. (1999). Comparison of knowledge and psychological well-being between patients with a short disease duration (≤ 1 year) and patients with more established rheumatoid arthritis (≥ 10 years duration). *Patient Education and Counseling, 38*, 195-203.

Barlow, J., Cullen, L., & Rowe, I. (2002). Educational preferences, psychological well-being and self-efficacy among people with rheumatoid arthritis. *Patient Education and Counseling, 46*, 11-19.

Barnabe, C., Elias, B., Bartlett, J., Roos, L., & Peschken, C. (2008). Arthritis in Aboriginal Manitobans: Evidence for a High Burden of Disease. *The Journal of rheumatology, 35*(6), 1145-1150.

Barrett-Connor, E. (1989). Epidemiology, obesity, and non-insulin-dependent diabetes mellitus. *Epidemiol Rev, 11*, 172.

Bartlett, J. (1998). The Medicine Wheel for comprehensive development in health. Unpublished Unpublished manuscript. University of Manitoba, Winnepeg.

Bates, C. E., & van Dam, C. H. (1984). Low incidence of schizophrenia in British Columbia coastal Indians. *Journal of Epidemiology and Community Health, 38*, 127-130.

BC FAS Resource Society (1998). *FAS Community Action Guide: Working Together for the Prevention of Fetal Alcohol Syndrome.*

Beals, J., Manson, S. M., Shore, J. H., Friedman, M., Ashcraft, M., Fairbank, J. A., et al. (2002). The Prevalence of Posttraumatic Stress Disorder Among American Indian Vietnam Veterans: Disparities and Context.

Journal of Traumatic Stress, 15(2), 89-97.

Beals, J., Novins, D. K., Spicer, P., Mitchell, C. M., & Manson, S. M. (2005). Prevalence of Mental Disorders and Utilization of Mental Health Services in Two American Indian Reservation Populations: Mental Health Disparities in a National Context. *American Journal of Psychiatry, 162*, 1723-1732.

Beauchamp, J., Blaauwbroek, M., Brulé, C., Campbell, J., Lava, J., Malone, L., et al. (2004). *Improving the Health of Canadians*. Ottawa: Canadian Institute of Health Information.

Beavis, M. A., Klos, N., Carter, T., & Douchant, C. (1997). Literature Review: Aboriginal Peoples and Homelessness. *Ottawa: Canada Mortgage and Housing Corporation*.

Bell, R., Smith, S., Arcury, T., Snively, B., Stafford, J., & Quandt, S. (2005). Prevalence and correlates of depressive symptoms among rural older African Americans, Native American, and Whites with diabetes. *Diabetes Care, 28*(4), 823-829.

Bennett, M., Blackstock, C., & De La Ronde, R. (2005). *A Literature Review and Annotated Bibliography on Aspects of Aboriginal Child Welfare in Canada 2nd Edition*: First Nations Research Site of the Centre of Excellence for Child Welfare and The First Nations Child & Family Caring Society of Canada.

Bernard, L., Lavallee, C., Gray-Donald, K., & Delisle, H. (1995). Overweight in Cree schoolchildren and adolescents associated with diet, low physical activity, and high television viewing. *J Am Diet Assoc, 95*(7), 800.

Black, R., Godwin, M., & Ponka, D. (2008). Breastfeeding among the Ontario James Bay Cree: a retrospective study. *Can J Public Health, 99*(2), 98-101.

Blackstock, C. (2005). Same Country: Same Lands, 78 Countries Away. *First Peoples Child & Family Review, 2*(1), 130-158.

Blackstock, C., Trochmé, N., & Bennett, M. (2004). Child Maltreatment Investigations Among Aboriginal and Non-Aboriginal Families in Canada. *Violence Against Women, 10*(8), 901-916.

Bobet, E. (1997). *Diabetes among First Nations People: Information from the 1991 Aboriginal Peoples Survey carried out by Statistics Canada* (Report). Ottawa: Medical Services Branch, Health Canada.

Bobet, E. (1998). Diabetes among First Nations people : information from the Statistics Canada 1991 Aboriginal Peoples Survey [microform .]. Ottawa: Health Canada.

Bohn, D. K. (2003). Lifetime Physical and Sexual Abuse, Substance Abuse, Depression, and Suicide Attempts Among Native American Women. *Issues in Mental Health Nursing, 24*(3), 333-352.

Boney, C. M., Verma, A., Tucker, R., & Vohr, B. R. (2005). Metabolic syndrome in childhood: association with birth weight, maternal obesity, and gestational diabetes mellitus. *Pediatrics, 115*(3), e290.

Boston, P., Jordon, S., MacNamara, E., Kozolanka, K., Bobbish-Rondeau, E., Iserhoff, H., et al. (1997). Using participatory action research to understand the meanings Aboriginal Canadians attribute to the rising incidence of diabetes. *Chronic Diseases in Canada, 18*(1).

Boswell, J. B., & Nienhuys, T. G. (1996). Patterns of persistent otitis media in the first year of life in aboriginal and non-aboriginal infants. *Ann Otol Rhinol Laryngol, 105*(11), 893-900.

Botha-Scheepers, S., Riyazi, N., Kroon, H., Scharloo, M., Houwing-Duistermaat, J., Slagboom, W., et al. (2006). Activity limitations in the lower extermities in patients with osteoarthritis: The modifying effects of illness perceptions and mental health *Osteoarthritis and Cartilage, 14*, 1104-1110.

Bowd, A. D. (2005). Otitis media: health and social consequences for aboriginal youth in Canada's north. *Int J Circumpolar Health, 64*(1), 5-15.

Boyce, W. T., & Keating, D. P. (2004). Should we intervene to improve childhood circumstances. In D. Kuh & Y. Ben-Shlomo (Eds.), *A life course approach to chronic disease epidemiology* (pp. 415-445). New York: Oxford University Press.

Brasfield, C. R. (2001). Residential School Syndrome. *BC Medical Journal, 43*(2), 78-81.

Breastfeeding Committee for Canada (2002). Breastfeeding Statement of the Breastfeeding Committee for Canada Retrieved January 10, 2008, from http://www.breastfeedingcanada.ca/html/webdoc5.html

Broadley, A. J. M., Korszun, A., Jones, C. J. H., & Frenneaux, M. P. (2002). Arterial endothelial function is impaired in treated depression. *Heart, 88*, 521-524.

Brown, M. L., Goldie, S. J., Draisma, G., Harford, J., & Lipscomb, J. (2006). Health Service Interventions for Cancer: Control in Developing Countries. In D. T. Jamison, J. G. Breman, A. R. Measham, G. Alleyne, M. Claeson, D. B. Evans, P. Jha, A. Mills & P. Musgrove (Eds.), *Disease Control Priorities in Developing Countries* (Vol. 2, pp. 569-589): Disease Control Priorities in Developing Countries

Bruce, N., Perez-Padilla, R., & Albalak, R. (2000). Indoor air pollution in developing countries: a major environmental and public health challenge. *Bulletin of the World Health Organization, 78*(9), 1078-1092.

Bruce, S. G., Kliewer, E., Young, T. K., Mayer, T., & Wajda, A. (2003). Diabetes among the Metis of Canada: Defining the Population, Estimating the Disease. *Canadian Journal of Diabetes, 27*, 442-448.

Burant, C. F., & American Diabetes Association (2004). *Medical management of type 2 diabetes* (5th ed.). Alexandria, Va.: American Diabetes Association.

Burke, H., Zautra, A., Schultz, A., Reich, J., & Davis, M. (2002). Arthritis. In A. Christensen & M. Antoni (Eds.), *Chronic Physical Disorders: Behavioral Medicine's Perspective*. Padstow, Cornwall: Blackwell Publishers.

Cadman, D., Boyle, M., Szatmari, P., & Offord, D. (1987). Chronic illness, disability and mental and social well-being: Findings of the Ontario Child Health Study. *Pediatrics, 79*(5), 805-813.

Cairns, R. B., Cairns, B. D., & Neckerman, H. J. (1989). Early school dropout: configurations and determinants. *Child Dev, 60*(6), 1437-1452.

Campaign 2000 (2006). Oh Canada! Too Many Children in Poverty for Too Long, from http://campaign2000.ca/rc/rc06/06_

C2000NationalReportCard.pdf

Canada (2005a). *Fetal alcohol spectrum disorder (FASD) : a framework for action.* from http://www.publichealth.gc.ca/fasd.

Canada (2005b). *Fetal Alcohol Syndrome.* from http://www.hc-sc.gc.ca/fnih-spni/famil/preg-gros/intro_e.html.

Canada (2006a). *Chapter 12: The Mental Health and Well-being of Aboriginal Peoples in Canada.* Ottawa: Minister of Public Works and Government Services Canada.

Canada (2006b). *Substance abuse issues and public policy in Canada: Canada's federal strategy.* from http://www.parl.gc.ca/information/library/PRBpubs/prb0615-e.html.

Canada, B. C. (2001). *The Health and Well-being of Aboriginal People in British Columbia.*

Canada. Parliament. House of Commons. Standing Committee on Health (1995). Towards holistic wellness, the Aboriginal peoples: report [microform]. Ottawa: The Standing Committee.

Canadian Arthritis Society (2004). *Revealing the impact of arthritis on the lives of Canadians.*

Canadian Cancer Society (2008, September). What is Cancer? Retrieved June, 2009, from http://www.cancer.ca/Canada-wide/About%20cancer/What%20is%20cancer.aspx?sc_lang=en

Canadian Institute for Health Information (2006). *How Healthy Are Rural Canadians?* from http://secure.cihi.ca/cihiweb/products/acknowledgements_rural_canadians_2006_report_e.pdf.

Canadian Institute for Health Information, Canadian Lung Association, Health Canada, & Statistics Canada (2001). *Respiratory Disease in Canada.*

Canadian Pediatric Society (2002). Fetal Alcohol Syndrome. *Paediatr Child Health, 7*(3), 161-174.

Cardinal, J. C., Schopflocher, D. P., Svenson, L. W., Morrison, K. B., & Laing, L. (2004). *First Nations in Alberta: A focus on health service use.* Edmonton: Alberta Health and Wellness.

Carroll, L., Cassidy, J., & Coté, P. (2000). The Saskatchewan health and back pain survey: The prevalence and factors associated with depressive symptomatology in Saskatchewan adults. *Canadian Journal of Public Health, 91*(6), 459-464.

Carson, B., Dunbar, T., Chenhall, R. D., & Bailie, R. (2007). *Social Determinants of Indigenous Health*. Crows Nest, NSW, Australia: Allen & Unwin.

Carver, C. (2007). Stress, Coping and Health. In H. Friedman & R. Cohen Silver (Eds.), *Foundations of Health Psychology*. Oxford: Oxford University Press.

Casey, P. (2001). Adult adjustment disorder: A review of its current diagnostic status. *Journal of Psychiatric Practice 7*(1), 32-40.

Casey, P., Maracy, M., Kelly, B., Lehtinen, V., Ayuso-Mateos, J., Dalgard, O., et al. (2006). Can adjustment disorder and depressive episode be distinguished? Results from ODIN. *Journal of Affective Disorders, 92*, 291-297.

Cassileth, B., Lusk, E., Strouse, T., Miller, D., Brown, L., Cross, P., et al. (1984). Psychosocial status in chronic illness. *The New England Journal of Medicine`, 311*(8), 506-511.

Caulfield, L. E., Harris, S. B., Whalen, E. A., & Sugamori, M. E. (1998). Maternal nutritional status, diabetes and risk of macrosomia among Native Canadian women. *Early Hum Dev, 50*(3), 293-303.

CBC News (2003). More chronic illness among off-reserve aboriginals: study, from http://www.cbc.ca/news/story/2003/09/24/aboriginal_statscan030924.html

Centre for Aboriginal Health Research (2009). *Global Indigenous Health Research Symposium Report. Papers and Presentations: Directions and Themes in International Indigenous Health Research 2008*. Victoria: University of Victoria.

Centres of Excellence for Children's Well-being (2008). Early Child Development Retrieved August 15, 2008, from http://www.excellence-jeunesenfants.ca/mission.asp?lang=EN

Chandler, M. J., & Lalonde, C. (1998). Cultural Continuity as a Hedge Against Suicide in Canada's First Nations. *Transcultural Psychiatry, 35*(2), 191-219.

Chansonneuve, D. (2005). *Reclaiming Connections: Understanding Residential School Trauma Among Aboriginal People.* Ottawa: Aboriginal Healing Foundation.

Chartrand, L. N. (2006). *Métis Residential School Participation: A Literature Review.* Ottawa: Aboriginal Healing Foundation.

Chrisjohn, R., & Young, S. (1995). *The Circle Game: Shadow and Substance in the Residential School Experience in Canada.* Penticton, BC.

Chronic Disease Prevention Alliance of Canada (2006). *A Call to Action from Conference Participants.* Paper presented at the Integrated Chronic Disease Prevention - *Building it Together.* from http://www.cdpac.ca/media.php?mid=270

CIHR (2007). *CIHR Guidelines for Health Research Involving Aboriginal Peoples.* from http://www.cihr-irsc.gc.ca/e/29134.html.

Clarke, H. F., Joseph, R., Deschamps, M., Hislop, T. G., Band, P. R., & Atleo, R. (1998). Reducing cervical cancer among First Nations women. *Can Nurse, 94*(3), 36-41.

Claussen, B., Davey Smith, G., & Thelle, D. (2003). Impact of childhood and adulthood socioeconomic position on cause specific mortality: the Oslo Mortality Study. *J Epidemiol Community Health., 57*(1), 40.

Cliver, S. P., Goldenberg, R. L., Cutter, G. R., Hoffman, H. J., Davis, R. O., & Nelson, K. G. (1995). The effect of cigarette smoking on neonatal anthropometric measurements. *Obstet Gynecol., 85*(4), 625-630.

Coates, H. L., Morris, P. S., Leach, A. J., & Couzos, S. (2002). Otitis media in Aboriginal children: tackling a major health problem. *Med J Aust, 177*(4), 177-178.

Condon, J. R., Barnes, T., Armstrong, B. K., Selva-Nayagam, S., & Elwood, J. M. (2005). Stage at diagnosis and cancer survival for Indigenous Australians in the Northern Territory. *Medical Journal of Australia, 182*(6), 277-280.

Cooke, M., Beavon, D. J. K., & McHardy, M. (2004). *Measuring the well-being of aboriginal people.* from http://www.ainc-inac.gc.ca/pr/ra/mwb/index_e.html

Corrado, R. R., Cohen, I. M., Aboriginal Healing Foundation (Canada), & Corrado Research and Evaluation Associates. (2003). *Mental health profiles for a sample of British Columbia's aboriginal survivors of the Canadian residential school system : prepared for the Aboriginal Healing Foundation.* Ottawa: Aboriginal Healing Foundation.

Cueller, J. (1990). *Aging and health: American Indian/Alaska native.* . Stanford, CA: Stanford Geratric Education Centre, Division of Family and Community Medicine.

Dabelea, D., Hanson, R. L., Lindsay, R. S., Pettitt, D. J., Imperatore, G., Gabir, M. M., et al. (2000). Intrauterine exposure to diabetes conveys risks for type 2 diabetes and obesity: a study of discordant sibships. *Diabetes, 49*(12), 2208-2211.

Dabelea, D., & Pettitt, D. J. (2001). Intrauterine diabetic environment confers risks for type 2 diabetes mellitus and obesity in the offspring, in addition to genetic susceptibility. *J Pediatr Endocrinol Metab, 14*(8), 1085-1091.

Damm, P. (2009). Future risk of diabetes in mother and child after gestational diabetes mellitus *International Journal of Gynecology & Obstetrics, 104*(Suppliment 1), S25-26.

Dangoor, N., & Florian, V. (1994). Women with chronic physical disabilities: Correlates of their long-term psychosocial adaptation. *International Journal of Rehabilitation Research, 17*(2), 159-168.

Daniel, M., Gamble, D., Henderson, J., & Burgess, S. (1995). Diabetes prevalence, behavioural and anthropometric risk factors, and psychosocial constructs in three Aboriginal communities in central British Columbia. *Chronic Diseases in Canada, 16*(4).

Daniel, M., O'Dea, K., Rowley, K. G., McDermott, R., & Kelly, S. (1999). Glycated hemoglobin as an indicator of social environmental stress among Indigenous versus Westernized populations. *Preventive Medicine, 29*, 405-413.

Daniel, M., Rowley, K. G., Herbert, C. P., O'Dea, K., & Green, L. W.

(2001). Lipids and psychosocial status in aboriginal persons with and at risk for Type 2 diabetes: Implications for tertiary prevention. *Patient Education and Counselling, 43*, 85-95.

Dappleton Research Team (2003). GVRD Aboriginal Homelessness Study 2003 (Abridged). In A. H. S. C. (AHSC) (Ed.). Vancouver: dappleton research.

Davidson, K., Kupfer, D., Bigger, T., Califf, R., Carney, R., Coyne, J., et al. (2006). Assessment and treatment of depression in patients with cardiovascular disease: National health, lung, and blood institute working group report. *Ann Behav Med, 32*(3), 121-126.

De Broucker, P., & Lavalee, L. (1998). "Intergenerational aspects of education and literacy skills acquisition." in M. Corak (ed.)Labour Markets, Social Institutions, and the Future of Canada's Children Available from http://www.cansim.net/english/freepub/89-553-XIB/89-553-XIB00098.pdf

de Groot, M., Anderson, R., Freedland, K., Clouse, R., & Lustman, P. (2001). Association of depression and diabetes complications: a meta-analysis. *Psychosomatic Medicine, 63*, 619-630.

De Marco, R. R. (2000). The epidemiology of major depression: implications of occurrence, recurrence, and stress in a Canadian community sample. *Can J Psychiatry, 45*(1), 67-74.

Dean, H. J., Mundy, R. L., & Moffatt, M. (1992). Non-insulin-dependent diabetes mellitus in Indian children in Manitoba. *CMAJ: Canadian Medical Association Journal, 147*(1), 52-57.

DeGagné, M. (2007). Toward an Aboriginal paradigm of healing: addressing the legacy of residential schools. *Australasian Psychiatry, 15*(Supplement), S49-S53.

Delisle, H. F., Rivard, M., & Ekoe, J. M. (1995). Prevalence estimates of diabetes and of other cardiovascular risk factors in the two largest Algonquin communities of Quebec. *Diabetes Care, 18*(9), 1255-1259.

Denny, C. H., D; Goins ,RT; Croft ,JB (2005). Disparities in chronic disease risk factors and health status between American Indian/Alaska Native and White elders: findings from a telephone survey, 2001 and 2002. [peer reviewed]. *American Journal Of Public Health, 95*(5), 825-827.

Deters, P. B., Novins, D. K., Fickenscher, A., & Beals, J. (2006). Trauma and Posttraumatic Stress Disorder Symptomatology: Patterns Among American Indian Adolescents in Substance Abuse Treatment. *American Journal of Orthopsychiatry, 76*(3), 335-345.

Dewailly, E., Blanchet, C., Lemieux, S., Sauve, L., Gingras, S., Ayotte, P., et al. (2001). n-3 Fatty acids and cardiovascular disease risk factors among the Inuit of Nunavik. *Am J Clin Nutr, 74*(4), 464-473.

Dickens, C., McGowan, L., Clark-Carter, D., & Creed, F. (2002). Depression in rheumatoid arthritis: A systemic review of the literature with meta-analysis. *Psychosomatic Medicine, 64*, 52-60.

Dictionary, C. M. O. R. O. (2002a). osteoarthritis Available from <http://www.oxfordreference.com/views/ENTRY.html?subview=Main&entry=t60.e9493>

Dictionary, C. M. O. R. O. (2002b). osteoporosis Available from <http://www.oxfordreference.com/views/ENTRY.html?subview=Main&entry=t60.e9493>

Dion Stout, M., & Harp, R. (2007). *Lump Sum Compensation Payments Research Project: The Circle Rechecks Itself - Draft*. Ottawa: Aboriginal Healing Foundation.

Dion Stout, M., & Kipling, G. (2003). *Aboriginal People, Resilience and the Residential School Legacy*. Ottawa: Aboriginal Healing Foundation.

Dorner, T., & Rieder, A. (2004). Risk management of coronary heart disease-prevention. *Wien Med Wochenschr, 154*(11-12), 257.

Dowrick, C. (2006). Chickens and eggs: Examining the links between mental health and chronic disease. *International Journal of Psychiatry in Medicince, 36*(3), 263-267.

Durie, M., Allan, G. R., & Cunningham, C. W. (1997). Oranga Kaumatua The Health and Wellbeing of Older Maori.

Dyck, R. F., Klomp, H., & Tan, L. (2001). From “thrifty genotype” to “hefty fetal phenotype”: the relationship between high birthweight and diabetes in Saskatchewan Registered Indians. *Can J Public Health, 92*(5),

340-344.

Dyck, R. F., Klomp, H., Tan, L. K., Turnell, R. W., & Boctor, M. A. (2002). A comparison of rates, risk factors, and outcomes of gestational diabetes between aboriginal and non-aboriginal women in the Saskatoon health district. *Diabetes Care, 25*(3), 487.

Ellickson, P. T., Joan; Klein, David J. (2001). High-risk behaviors associated with early smoking: results from a 5-year follow-up*1 *Journal of Adoloescent health, 28*(6), 465-473.

Encyclopædia Britannica (2006). rheumatism. Retrieved 11 Dec: <http://search.eb.com/eb/article-9063420>.

Epstein, R. (1982). Letters to the Editor. *Can J Public Health, 73*, 433-434.

Evers, A., Kraaimaat, F., Geenen, R., & Bijlsma, J. (1997). Determinants of psychological distress and its course in the first year after diagnosis in Rheumatoid Arthritis patients. *Journal of Behavioral Medicine, 20*(5), 489-504.

Fava, M., & Kendler, K. (2000). Major depressive disorder. *Neuron, 28*, 335-341.

First Nations and Inuit Health Branch (2000/2001). Mortality rate for lung cancer, prostate cancer, breast cancer, colorectal cancer, acute myocardial infarction (AMI) and stroke (Age-standardized to the 1991 Canadian population): Health Canada.

First Nations and Inuit Regional Health Survey National Steering Committee (1999). *First Nations and Inuit Regional Health Survey National Report 1999*: First Nations and Inuit Regional Health Survey National Steering Committee.

First Nations Centre (2004). First Nations and Inuit Regional Health Surveys, 1997 : A synthesis of the national and regional reports. Ottawa: First Nations Centre at the National Aboriginal Health Organization. .

First Nations Centre (2005). First Nations Regional Longitudinal Health Survey (RHS) 2002/2003: Results for Adults, Youth and Children Living in First Nations Communities. Ottawa: First Nations Centre at the National Aboriginal Health Organization. .

Folsom, D. P., Hawthorne, W., Lindamer, L., Gilmer, T., Bailey, A., Golshan, S., et al. (2005). Prevalence and Risk Factors for Homelessness and Utilization of Mental Health Services Among 10,340 Patients with Serious Mental Illness in a Large Public Mental Health System. *American Journal of Psychiatry, 162*, 370-376.

Fournier, S., & Crey, E. (1997). *Stolen From Our Embrace: The Abduction of First Nations Children and the Restoration of Aboriginal Communities.* Vancouver: Douglas & McIntyre Ltd.

Frank, S. (1992). *Family Violence in Aboriginal Communities: A First Nations Report.* Victoria, B.C.: Minister of Women's Equality.

Franks, P. W., Looker, H. C., Kobes, S., Touger, L., Tataranni, P. A., Hanson, R. L., et al. (2006). Gestational glucose tolerance and risk of type 2 diabetes in young Pima Indian offspring. *Diabetes, 55*(2), 460-465.

Frasure-Smith, N., & Lesperance, F. (2005). Reflections on depression as a cardiac risk factor. *Psychosomatic Medicine, 67*, S19-S25.

Gallagher, R. P., & Elwood, J. M. (1979). Cancer mortality among Chinese, Japanese, and Indians in British Columbia, 1964-73. *Natl Cancer Inst Monogr*(53), 89-94.

Gask, L. (2005). Is depression a chronic illness? For the motion. *Chronic Illness, 1*, 101-106.

Gaudette, L. A., Freitag, S., Dufour, R., Baikie, M., Gao, R. N., & Wideman, M. (1996). Cancer in Circumpolar Inuit. Background information for cancer patterns in Canadian Inuit. *Acta Oncol, 35*(5), 527-533.

Geyorfi-Dyke, E. (2008). Poverty and Chronic Disease: Recommendations for Action. In Chronic Disease Prevention Alliance of Canada (Ed.): CDPAC.

Ghadirian, P. (2005). *Sleeping With A Killer.* from http://www.hc-sc.gc.ca/hl-vs/pubs/tobac-tabac/swk-dat/index_e.html.

Gilmer, T., O'Conner, P., Rush, W., Crain, L., Whitebird, R., Hanson, A., et al. (2005). Predictors of health care costs in adults with diabetes. *Diabetes Care, 28*(1), 59-64.

Glassman, A., & Shapiro, P. (1998). Depression and the course of coronary artery disease. *Am J Psychiatry, 155*(1), 4-11.

Goldney, R., Phillips, P., Fisher, L., & Wilson, D. (2004). Diabetes, depression, and quality of life: A population study. *Diabetes Care, 27*(5), 1066-1070.

Gonder-Frederisk, L., Cox, D., & Clarke, W. (2002). Diabetes. In A. Christensen & M. Antoni (Eds.), *Chronic Physical Disorders: Behavioral Medicine's Perspective.* Cornwall: Blackwell Publishers.

Goodman, A. (1990). Addiction: definition and implications. *British Journal of Addiction, 85*, 1403-1408.

Government of Canada (2003). *Report of the Auditor General to the House of Commons.* Retrieved August 13, 2008. from http://www.oag-bvg.gc.ca/internet/English/aud_ch_oag_200304_6_e_12912.html.

Graham, H., & Power, C. (2004). Childhood disadvantage and health inequalities: a framework for policy based on lifecourse research. *Child: care, health and development, 30*(6), 671.

Grams, G. D., Herbert, C., Heffernan, C., Calam, B., Wilson, M. A., Grzybowski, S., et al. (1996). Haida perspectives on living with non-insulin-dependent diabetes. *CMAJ: Canadian Medical Association Journal, 155*(11), 1563-1568.

Grange, J., Story, A., & Zumla, A. (2001). Tuberculosis in disadvantaged groups. *Current Opinion in Pulmonary Medicine, 7*(3), 160.

Gray, W. (2005). Young People and... Cancer!?, from http://www.ayn.ca/ViewNews.aspx?id=366

Green, C., Blanchard, J. F., Young, T. K., & Griffith, J. (2003). The epidemiology of diabetes in the Manitoba-registered First Nation population: current patterns and comparative trends. *Diabetes Care, 26*(7), 1993-1998.

Green, C., Hoppa, R., Young, T. K., & Blanchard, J. F. (2003). Geographic analysis of diabetes prevalence in an urban area. *Social Science & Medicine,*

57(3), 551-560.

Greene, C., Blanchard, J., & Wajda, A. (1999). Projecting future diabetes prevalence in Manitoba First Nations *Proceedings of the 4th International Conference on Diabetes and Indigenous People, San Diego, 1997.* Tucson, Arizona: Native American Research and Training Center, University of Arizona.

Greer, J. R., Abbey, D. E., & Burchette, R. J. (1993). Asthma related to occupational and ambient air pollutants in nonsmokers. *J Occup Med, 35*(9), 909-915.

Hales, C. N., & Barker, D. J. (1992). Type 2 (non-insulin-dependent) diabetes mellitus: the thrifty phenotype hypothesis. *Diabetologia, 35*(7), 595-601.

Hammen, C. (1997). *Depression*. Padstow, Cornwall: Psychology Press Ltd.

Hanley, A., Harris, S., Mamakeesick, M., Goodwin, K., Fiddler, E., Hegele, R., et al. (2005). Complications of Type 2 diabetes among Aboriginal Canadians. *Diabetes Care, 28*(8), 2054-2057.

Hanley, A. J., Harris, S. B., Gittelsohn, J., Wolever, T. M., Saksvig, B., & Zinman, B. (2000). Overweight among children and adolescents in a Native Canadian community: prevalence and associated factors. *Am J Clin Nutr., 71*(3), 693.

Harper, S. (2008, June 11). Prime Minister Harper offers full apology on behalf of Canadians for the Indian Residential Schools system, from http://pm.gc.ca/eng/media.asp?id=2149

Harris, S. B., Caulfield, L. E., Sugamori, M. E., Whalen, E. A., & Henning, B. (1997). The epidemiology of diabetes in pregnant Native Canadians. A risk profile. *Diabetes Care, 20*(9), 1422-1425.

Harris, S. B., Gittelsohn, J., Hanley, A., Barnie, A., Wolever, T. M., Gao, J., et al. (1997). The prevalence of NIDDM and associated risk factors in native Canadians. *Diabetes Care, 20*(2), 185-187.

Harris, S. B., Glazier, R., Eng, K., & McMurray, L. (1998). Disease patterns among Canadian aboriginal children. Study in a remote rural setting. *Canadian Family Physician, 44*, 1869-1877.

Harris, S. B., Perkins, B. A., & Whalen-Brough, E. (1996). Non-insulin-dependent diabetes mellitus among First Nations children. New entity among First Nations people of north western Ontario. *Can Fam Physician, 42*, 869-876.

Harris, S. B., Zinman, B., Hanley, A., Gittelsohn, J., Hegele, R., Connelly, P. W., et al. (2002). The impact of diabetes on cardiovascular risk factors and outcomes in a native Canadian population. *Diabetes Res Clin Pract, 55*(2), 165.

Hawley, D., & Wolfe, F. (1993). Depression is not more common in rheumatoid arthritis: A 10 year longitudinal study of 6,153 patients with rheumatoid arthritis. *The Journal of Rheumatology, 20*, 2025-2031.

Health Canada (1994). Mercury and Human Health.

Health Canada (1999). *Diabetes in Canada: National Statistics and Opportunities for Improved Surveillance, Prevention, and Control* (Report). Ottawa: Centre for Chronic Disease Prevention and Control, Health Canada.

Health Canada (2000a). Chapter 7: Breastfeeding *Family-Centred Maternity and Newborn Care: National Guidelines.* Ottawa.

Health Canada (2000b). *Diabetes among Aboriginal People in Canada: The evidence.* from http://www.hc-sc.gc.ca/fnih-spni/pubs/diabete/2001_evidence_faits/index_e.html

Health Canada (2000c). *Diabetes in Canada, national statistics and opportunities for improved surveillance, prevention and control.*

Health Canada (2002). *A Report on Mental Illnesses in Canada.* from http://www.phac-aspc.gc.ca/publicat/miic-mmac/pdf/men_ill_e.pdf

Health Canada (2003a). *Arthritis in Canada. An ongoing challenge.*

Health Canada (2003b). *Smoking in Canada:.*

Health Canada (2003c). *The statistical profile on Health of First Nations in Canada.* Ottawa: Health Canada, First Nations and Inuit Health Branch.

Health Canada (2005a). *A statistical profile on the health of First Nations in Canada for the year 2000.* from www.healthcanada.gc.ca/FNHealthStats

Health Canada (2005b). *The statistical profile on the health of First Nations in Canada for the year of 2000.*

Health Canada (2009). First Nations and Inuit Health Fact Sheet.

Heaman, M. I., & Chalmers, K. (2005). Prevalence and correlates of smoking during pregnancy: a comparison of aboriginal and non-aboriginal women in manitoba. *Birth, 32*(4), 299-305.

Helgeson, V., & Reynolds, K. (2002). Social psychological aspects of chronic disease In A. Christensen & M. Antoni (Eds.), *Chronic Physical Disorders: Behavioral Medicine's Perspective.* Padstow, Cornwall: Blackwell Publishers.

Helin, S. (2002). Aboriginal Homelessness, Prince Rupert and Port Edward: An Assets and Gap Review of Existing Services for the Homeless. Prince Rupert: Prince Rupert Steering Committee on Aboriginal Homelessness.

Hippisley-Cox, J., Fielding, K., & Pringle, M. (1998). Depression as a risk factor for ischaemic heart disease in men: population based case-control study. *BMJ, 316*, 1714-1719.

Hirsch, R., Fernandes, R. J., Pillemer, S. R., Hochberg, M. C., Lane, N. E., Altman, R. D., et al. (1998). Hip osteoarthritis prevalence estimates by three radiographic scoring systems. *Arthritis Rheum, 41*(2), 361-368.

Hod, M. (2003). *Textbook of diabetes and pregnancy.* London ; New York; Independence, KY: Martin Dunitz; Distributed in the USA by Taylor & Francis.

Horsten, M., Mittleman, M., Wamala, S., Schenck-Gustafsson, & Orth-Gomér, K. (2000). Depressive symptoms and lack of social integration in relation to prognosis of CHD in middle-aged women: The Stockholm Female Coronary Risk Study. *European Heart Journal, 21*(1072-80).

Hu, G., & Ran, P. (2009). Indoor Air Pollution as a Lung Health Hazard: Focus on Populous Countries. *Current Opinion in Pulmonary Medicine, 15*(2), 158-164.

Hubert, H. B., Feinleib, M., McNamara, P. M., & Castelli, W. P. (1983). Obesity as an independent risk factor for cardiovascular disease: a 26-year follow-up of participants in the Framingham Heart Study. *Circulation, 67*(5), 968-977.

Hull, J., Research, Analysis, D., & Indian and Northern Affairs, C. (2000). *Aboriginal Post-secondary Education and Labour Market Outcomes Canada, 1996*: Research & Analysis Directorate, Indian and Northern Affairs Canada.

Humphrey, M., & Holzheimer, D. (2000). A prospective study of gestation and birthweight in Aboriginal pregnancies in far north Queensland. *Aust N Z J Obstet Gynaecol, 40*(3), 326-330.

Hwang, S. W. (2001). Homelessness and health. *Canadian Medical Association Journal, 164*(2), 229-233.

Hwang, S. W., & Bugeja, A. L. (2000). Barriers to appropriate diabetes management among homeless people in Toronto. *Canadian Medical Association Journal, 163*(2), 161-165.

Hysing, M., Elgen, I., Gillberg, C., Lie, S. A., & Lundervold, A. J. (2007). Chronic physical illness and mental health in children. Results from a large-scale population study. *Journal of Child Psychology and Psychiatry, 48*(8), 785–792.

ICD-10, I. C. o. D. (2006). Diseases of musculoskeletal and connective tissue. Retrieved 5 Dec2006: http://www.who.int/classifications/apps/icd/icd10online/

ICD-10. International Classification of Diseases (2006). Diseases of musculoskeletal and connective tissue. Retrieved 5 Dec2006: http://www.who.int/classifications/apps/icd/icd10online/

INAC Measuring Inuit Wellbeing. Retrieved from http://www.ainc-inac.gc.ca/ai/rs/pubs/re/miwb/miwb-eng.pdf

INAC (2004). *Measuring First Nations well-being.*

Indian and Northern Affairs (2005). First Nations Housing Retrieved August 13, 2008, from http://www.ainc-inac.gc.ca/pr/info/info104_e.html

Isaak, C. A., & Marchessault, G. (2008). Meaning of health: The perspectives of Aboriginal adults and youth in a northern Manitoba First

Nations community. *Canadian Journal of Diabetes, 32*(2), 114-122.

Jackson-Triche, M., Sullivan, J. G., Wells, K., Rogers, W., Camp, P., & Mazel, R. (2000). Depression and health-related quality of life in ethnic minorities seeking care in general medical settings. *Journal of Affective Disorders, 58*, 89-97.

Jackson, D. J., Batiste, E., & Rendall-Mkosi, K. (2007). Effect of smoking and alcohol use during pregnancy on the occurrence of low birthweight in a farming region in South Africa. *Paediatric and Perinatal Epidemiology, 21*(5), 432-440.

Jacobson, A. M., De Groot, M., & Samson, J. A. (1994). The evaluation of two measures of quality of life in patients with Type I and Type II diabetes. *Diabetes Care, 17*(4), 267-274.

Jacobson, A. M., de Groot, M., & Samson, J. A. (1997). The effects of psychiatric disorders and symptoms on quality of life in patients with Type I and Type II diabetes mellitus. *Quality of Life Research, 6*, 11-20.

Jacono, J., Jacono, B., Cano, P., Segami, M., & Rubin, L. (1996). An epidemiological study of rheumatoid arthritis in a northern Ontario clinical practice: the role of ethnicity. *J Adv Nurs, 24*(1), 31-35.

Jin, A., Martin, J. D., & Sarin, C. (2002). Diabetes mellitus in the First Nations population of British Columbia, Canada. Part 2. Hospital morbidity. *International Journal of Circumpolar Health, 61*(3), 254-259.

Jones, R., Yates, W., Williams, S., Zhou, M., & Hardman, L. (1999). Outcome for adjustment disorder for depressed mood: comparison with other mood disorders. *Journal of Affective Disorders, 55*, 55-61.

Kaijser, M., Edstedt Bonamy, A. K., Akre, O., Cnattingius, S., Granath, F., Norman, M., et al. (2009). Perinatal Risk Factors for Diabetes in Later Life. *Diabetes, 58*(3), 523-526.

Kasprow, W. J., & Rosenheck, R. A. (1998). Substance Use and Psychiatric Problems of Homeless Native American Veterans. *Psychiatric Services, 49*(3), 345-350.

Katon, W., & Sullivan, M. (1990). Depression and chronic medical illness. *Journal of Clinical Psychiatry, 51*(6 (Suppl)), 3-11.

Kee, C. (2003). Older adults with osteoarthritis: Psychological status and physical function. *Journal of Gerontological Nursing, 29*(12), 26-34.

King, D. (2006). *A Brief Report of The Federal Government of Canada's Residential School System for Inuit.* Ottawa: Aboriginal Healing Foundation.

Kirmayer, L., Brass, G., & Tait, C. (2000). The mental health of Aboriginal peoples: Transformations of identity and community. *Canadian Journal of Psychiatry, 45*, 607-615.

Kirmayer, L., Fletcher, C., Corin, E., & Boothroyd, L. (1994). *Inuit Concepts of Mental Health and Illness: An Ethnographic Study.*

Kirmayer, L., Simpson, C., & Cargo, M. (2003). Healing traditions: culture, community and mental health promotion with Canadian Aboriginal peoples. *Australasian Psychiatry, 11*(Supplement), S15-S23.

Kliewer, E., Mayer, T., & Wajda, A. (2002). The Health of Manitoba's Métis Population and their Utilization of Medical Services: A Pilot Study: Winnipeg: Cancer Care Manitoba and Manitoba Health.

Knol, M., Twisk, J., Beekman, A. T. F., Heine, R., Snoek, F., & Pouwer, F. (2006). Depression as a risk factor for the onset of type 2 diabetes mellitus. A meta-analysis. *Diabetologia, 49*, 837-845.

Kramer, J., Harker, J., & Wong, A. (2002). Arthritis beliefs and self-care in an urban American Indian population. *Arthritis & Rheumatism, 47*(6), 588-594.

Kuh, D., & Ben-Shlomo, Y. (Eds.). (2004). *A Life Course approach to Chronic Disease Epidemiology* (2nd Ed. ed.). New York: Oxford University Press.

Kumanyika, S. (1993). Ethnicity and obesity development in children. *Ann N Y Acad Sci., 699*, 81.

Lagacé, C., Perruccio, A., DesMeules, M., & Badley, E. (2003). The Impact of Arthritis on Canadians *Arthritis in Canada: An ongoing challenge*: Health Canada.

Lawrence, R. C., Helmick, C. G., Arnett, F. C., Deyo, R. A., Felson, D. T., Giannini, E. H., et al. (1998). Estimates of the prevalence of arthritis and selected musculoskeletal disorders in the United States. *Arthritis & Rheumatism 41*(5), 778-799.

Leach, A. J. (1999). Otitis media in Australian Aboriginal children: an overview. *Int J Pediatr Otorhinolaryngol, 49 Suppl 1*, S173-178.

Lee, K. K. (2000). Urban Poverty in Canada: A Statistical Profile, from http://www.ccsd.ca/pubs/2000/up/

Lefley, H. P. (1990). Culture and Chronic Mental Illness. *Hospital and Community Psychiatry, 41*(3), 277-286.

Leslie, W. D., Derksen, S., Prior, H. L., Lix, L. M., Metge, C., & O'Neil, J. (2006). The interaction of ethnicity and chronic disease as risk factors for osteoporotic fractures: a comparison in Canadian Aboriginals and non-Aboriginals. *Osteoporosis Int, 17*, 1358-1368.

Lesperance, F., Frasure-Smith, N., & Talajic, M. (1996). Major depression before and after myocardial infarction: Its nature and consequences. *Psychosomatic Medicine, 58*, 99-110.

Lidgren, L. (2003). The Bone and Joint Decade 2000-2010. *Bulletin of the WHO,* (81), 629

Linscott, R. J., Marie, D., Arnott, K. L., & Clark, B. L. (2006). Over-representation of Maori New Zealanders among adolescents in a schizotypy taxon. *Schizophrenia Research, 84*, 289-296.

Logan, T. E. (2001). *Lost Generations: The Silent Métis of the Residential School System - Revised Interim Report*. Ottawa: Aboriginal Healing Foundation.

Mackinko, B., Starfield, B., & Shi, L. (2003). The contribution of primary care systems to health outcomes within Organization for Economic Cooperation and Development (OECD) countries, 1970-1998. *HSR: Health Services Research, 38*, 831-865.

MacMillan, H. L., MacMillan, A. B., Offord, D. R., & Dingle, J. L. (1996). Aboriginal Health. [review]. *Canadian Medical Association Journal, 155*(11), 1569 - 1578.

Malatest, R. A. (2004). Aboriginal Peoples and Post-Secondary Education: What Educators Have Learned. Montreal, QC: Canada Millennium Scholarship Foundation.

Marmot, M. G. (2005). Social determinants of health inequalities. *The*

Lancet, 365(9464), 1099-1104.

Marmot, M. G., & Wilkinson, R. G. (1999). *Social Determinants of Health.* New York: Oxford University Press.

Marrett, L. D., & Chaudhry, M. (2003). Cancer incidence and mortality in Ontario First Nations, 1968-1991 (Canada). [Cohort study]. *Cancer Causes and Control, 14*(3), 259 - 268.

Marrett, L. D., Jones, C. R., & Wishart, K. (2004). *First Nations Cancer research and Surveillance priorities for Canada.* Ottawa: Cancer Care.

Martin, B. D., & Macdonald, S. M. (1998). The management of ear disease: guidelines for Aboriginal health care programs. *Int J Circumpolar Health, 57 Suppl 1*, 268-275.

Matthews, D. D. (2003). *Diabetes sourcebook.* Detroit: Omnigraphics.

Maxim, P. S., White, J. P., Whitehead, P. C., & Beavon, D. (2000). An analysis of wage and income inequality - Dispersion and polarization of income among Aboriginal and non-Aboriginal Canadians. . London: University of Western Ontario.

Mayor's Homelessness Action Task Force (1999). Taking Responsibility for Homelessness. Toronto: City of Toronto.

Mayou, R., Bryant, B., & Turner, R. (1990). Quality of life in non-insulin-dependent diabetes and a comparison with insulin-dependent diabetes. *Journal of Psychosomatic Research, 34*(1), 1-11.

McCubbin, H., Thompson, E., Thompson, A., McCubbin, M., & Kaston, A. (1993). Culture, ethnicity, and the family: Critical factors in childhood chronic illnesses and disabilities. *Pediatrics, 91*(5), 1063-1070.

McEwan, B., & Swan, N. (1998). Good stress and bad stress. Mastering the control factor. part three. *The health report,* 2007

McEwen, B. S. (2006). Protective and damaging effects of stress mediators: Central role of the brain. *Dialogues Clin Neurosci, 8*(4), 367-381.

McIntyre, L. (2003). Food Security: More Than a Determinant of Health. *POLICY, 47*, 46.

McIntyre, L., & Shah, C. P. (1986). Prevalence of hypertension, obesity and smoking in three Indian communities in northwestern Ontario. *CMAJ: Canadian Medical Association Journal, 134*(4), 345-349.

Med-Help (2004, March 4). Ear Infection: Otitis Media. *Medical Library* Retrieved July 19, 2005, from http://www.med-help.net/OtitisMedia.html

Mendelson, M. (2004). *Aboriginal people in Canada's labour market: work and unemployment, today and tomorrow.* (Vol. 1). Ottawa: The Caledon institute of social policy.

Métis National Council (2006). Preliminary Assessment of Diabetes Programs for Métis Peoples

Mohamed, N., & Dooley, J. (1998). Gestational diabetes and subsequent development of NIDDM in aboriginal women of northwestern Ontario. *Int J Circumpolar Health, 57 Suppl 1*, 355-358.

Mohsin, M., Bauman, A. E., & Jalaludin, B. (2005). The Influence of antenatal and maternal factors on stillbirths and neonatal deaths in New South Wales, Austarlia. *Journal of Biosoc. Sci.*

Moore, V. M., & Davies, M. J. (2005). Diet during pregnancy, neonatal outcomes and later health. *Reprod Fertil Dev 17*(3), 341.

Moran, D. J., Waterford, J. E., Hollows, F., & Jones, D. L. (1979). Ear disease in rural Australia. *Med J Aust, 2*(4), 210-212.

Morris, K. (2007). (A Literature Review) Re-examining issues behind the loss of family and cultural and the impact on Aboriginal youth suicide rates. *First Peoples Child & Family Review, 3*(1), 133-142.

Morris, P. S. (1998). A systematic review of clinical research addressing the prevalence, aetiology, diagnosis, prognosis and therapy of otitis media in Australian Aboriginal children. *J Paediatr Child Health, 34*(6), 487-497.

Mowry, B., Lennon, D., & De Felice, C. (1994). Diagnosis of schizophrenia in a matched sample of Australian aborigines. *Acta Psychiatr Scand, 90*, 337-341.

Murray, W. (1994). *Environmental health: Risks posed by PCBs.*

Mussell, B., Cardiff, K., & White, J. (2004). *The Mental Health and Well-Being of Aboriginal Children and Youth: Guidance for New Approaches and*

Services. Chilliwack, BC: The Sal'i'shan Institute.

Nagyoca, I., Stewart, R., Macejova, Z., van Dijk, J., & van de Heuval, W. (2005). The impact of pain on psychological well-being in rheumatoid arthritis: The mediating effects of self-esteem and adjustment to disease. *Patient Education and Counseling, 58*, 55-62.

Nair, L., Nair, M. K. C., & Chacko, D. S. (2009). Markers of Fetal Onset Adult Diseases. *Indian Pediatrics, 46*(Suppliment), S48-54.

National Cancer Institute (2002). Alcohol and Cancer. from US National Institutes of Health: http://progressreport.cancer.gov/doc_detail.asp?pid=1&did=2005&chid=21&coid=206&mid=

National Native Addictions Partnership Foundation Inc. (2000). *NNADAP Renewal Framework For Implementing the Strategic Recommendations of the 1998, General Review of the National Native Alcohol and Drug Abuse Program.*

Newbold, K. B. (1998). Problems in search of solutions: health and Canadian Aboriginals. *J Community Health, 23*(1), 59-73.

Newman, S. (1997). Rheumatoid Arthritis. In A. Baum, S. Newman, J. Weinman, R. West & C. McManus (Eds.), *Cambridge Handbook of Psychology, Health and Medicine.* Cambridge: Cambridge University Press.

Nicholas, J., & Chen, Z. (2002). Osteoporosis in Native Americans *The IHS Primary Care Provider, May*, 94-101.

Nielsen, N. H., Storm, H. H., Gaudette, L. A., & Lanier, A. P. (1996). Cancer in the Circumpolar Inuit 1969-1988. [Summary]. *Acta Oncologica, 35*(5), 621-628.

NSW Health (2006). Chronic Diseases in Aboriginal Communities. *Aboriginal Chronic Care Program* Retrieved August 15, 2008, from http://www.health.nsw.gov.au/health_pr/avhp/approach.html

O'Keeffe, N., & Ranjith, G. (2007). Depression, demoralisation or adjustment disorder? Understanding emotional distress in the severely medically ill. *Clinical Medicine, 7*(5), 478-481.

O'Neil, J., Reading, J., Bartlett, J., Young, T. K., & Kaufert, J. (1999). Integrating a focus on Aboriginal health reserach in the development of the Canadian Institutes of Health Research: a concept paper. Unpublished Unpublished Manuscript. CIHR.

O'Neil, J. D. (2001). Chisasibi Housing and Health Report. Montreal, Que.: Grand COuncil of the Crees [Eeyou Istchee].

O'Neill, J. (2007, April 27, 2007). Senate committee chastises Canada for its treatment of aboriginal children. *Ottawa Citizen*. from http://www.canadiancrc.com/Newspaper_Articles/Ottawa_Citizen_Senate_Committee_chastises_Canada_treatment_aboriginal_children_27APR07.aspx.

Oberle, P. R., & INAC (1993). *The incidence of family poverty on Canadian Indian reserves*. Ottawa: Indian and Northern Affairs Canada.

Okada, S., Ichiki, K., Tanokuchi, S., Ishii, K., Hamada, H., & Ota, Z. (1995). Improvement of stress reduces glycated hemoglobin levels in patients with type 2 diabetes. *Journal of International Medical Research, 23*, 119-122.

Ong, M., & Weeramanthri, T. (2002). Stress and worry are central issues for indigenous heart attack survivors in the Northern Territory. *Australian Journal of Primary Health, 8*(2), 17-20.

Ontario Federation of Indian Friendship Centres (2004). Urban Aboriginal Child Poverty Background Retrieved July 21, 2008, from http://www.ofifc.org/ofifchome/page/notes.htm

Ontario Program for Optimal Therapeutics (2000). *Ontario drug therapy guidelines for stable ischemic heart disease in primary care.*

Ormel, J., Kempen, G. I. J. M., Penninx, B. W. J. H., Brilman, E. I., Beekman, A. T. F., & Van Sonderen, E. (1997). Chronic medical conditions and mental health in older people: disability and psychosocial resources mediate specific mental health effects. *Psychological Medicine, 27*, 1065-1077.

Orr, P., McDonald, S., Milley, D., & Brown, R. (2001). Bronchiolitis in Inuit children from a Canadian central arctic community, 1995-1996. *Int J Circumpolar Health, 60*(4), 649-658.

Paci, C. D. J., Dickson, C., Nickels, S., & Furgal, C. (2004). *Food Security of Northern Indigenous Peoples in a Time of Uncertainty.* Paper presented at the The Resilient North - Human Responses to Global Change. from http://www.nrf.is/Publications/The%20Resilient%20North/Plenary%204/3rd%20NRF_Plenary%204_PP_Paci%20et%20al.pdf

Palacio-Quintin, E. (2000). Les services de garde et le developpement de l'enfant. *ISUMA-Canadian Journal of Policy Research/Revue canadienne de recherche sur les politiques, 1*(2), 25-30.

Parker, G. (2005). Is depression a chronic illness? Parker opposes the motion. *Chronic Illness, 1*, 107-112.

Patten, S. (1999). Long-term medical conditions and major depression in the Canadian population. *Canadian Journal of Psychiatry, 44*, 151-157.

Penninx, B. W. J. H., Beekman, A. T. F., Ormel, J., Kriegsman, D., Boeke, J., van Eijk, J., et al. (1996). Psychological status among elderly people with chronic diseases: Does type of disease play a part? *Journal of Psychosomatic Research, 40*(5), 521-534.

Penninx, B. W. J. H., Leveille, S., Ferrucci, L., van Eijk, J., & Guralnik, J. (1999). Exploring the effect of depression on physical disability: Longitudinal evidence from the established populations for epidemiologic studies for the elderly. *American Journal of Public Health, 89*(9), 1346-1352.

Peschken, C. A., & Esdaile, J. M. (1999). Rheumatic diseases in North America's Indigenous peoples. *Seminars in Arthritis and Rheumatism, 28*(6), 368-391.

Pettitt, D. J. (1998). Gestational diabetes mellitus: who to test. How to test. *Diabetes Care, 21*(11), 1789.

Peyrot, M., & Rubin, R. (1997). Levels and risks of depression and anxiety symptomatology among diabetic adults. *Diabetes Care, 20*(4), 585-590.

PHAC (2004). Special Report of the Canadian Tuberculosis Committee - Tuberculosis Among the Aboriginal Peoples of Canada, 2000 to 2004 Retrieved June, 2009, from http://www.phac-aspc.gc.ca/publicat/2007/tbcan04/tbaboriginal-eng.php

Plumb, J. D. (2000). Homelessness: reducing health disparities, *Canadian Medical Association Journal* (Vol. 163, pp. 172-173): Can Med Assoc.

Pratt, L., Ford, D., Crum, R., Armenian, H., Gallo, J., & Eaton, W. (1996). Depression, psychotropic medication and risk of myocardial infarction: Prospective data from the Baltimore ECA follow-up. *Circulation, 94*, 3123-3129.

Prince, M., Patel, V., Saxena, S., Maj, M., Maselko, J., Phillips, M. R., et al. (2007). No health without mental health. *Lancet, 370*(9590), 859-877.

Quintero, G. (2000). "The lizard in the green bottle": "aging out" of problem drinking among Navajo men. *Social Science & Medicine, 51*, 1031-1045.

Rasmussen, C., Horne, K., & Witol, A. (2006). Neurobehavioral Functioning in Children with Fetal Alcohol Spectrum Disorder. *Child Neuropsychology, 12*, 453-468.

Reading, J. (1999). *An Examination of Residential Schools and Elder Health.* Ottawa: The Assembly of First Nations Resource Centre.

Reilly, J. J., Armstrong, J., Dorosty, A. R., Emmett, P. M., Ness, A., Rogers, I., et al. (2005). Early life risk factors for obesity in childhood: cohort study. *BMJ (Clinical research ed.), 330*(7504), 1357.

Retnakaran, R., Hanley, A. J. G., Connelly, P. W., Harris, S. B., & Zinman, B. (2005). Cigarette smoking and cardiovascular risk factors among Aboriginal Canadian youths. *Canadian Medical Association Journal, 173*(8), 885-889.

Ritchie, A. J., & Reading, J. L. (2004). Tobacco smoking status among Aboriginal youth. *Int J Circumpolar Health, 63 Suppl 2*, 405-409.

Roberts, R. A., & Roberts-Thomson, P. J. (1999). Rheumatic diseases in the Australian Aborigine. *Ann Rheum Dis 58*, 266-270.

Robin, R. W., Chester, B., Rasmussen, J. K., Jaranson, J. M., & Goldman, D. (1997). Prevalence and Characteristics of Trauma and Posttraumatic Stress Disorder in a Southwestern American Indian Community. *American Journal of Psychiatry, 154*(11), 1582-1588.

Robin, R. W., Gottesman, I. I., Albaugh, B., & Goldman, D. (2007). Schizophrenia and psychotic symptoms in families of two American Indian tribes. *BMC Psychiatry, 7*(30).

Rodrigues, S., Robinson, E. J., Kramer, M. S., & Gray-Donald, K. (2000). High rates of infant macrosomia: a comparison of a Canadian native and a non-native population. *J Nutr, 130*(4), 806-812.

Rosemann, T., Backenstrass, M., Joest, K., Rosemann, A., Szecsenyi, J., & Laux, G. (2007). Predictors of depression in a sample of 1,021 primary care patients with osteoarthritis. *Arthritis & Rheumatism, 57*(3), 415-422.

Rosenberg, T., & Martel, S. (1998). Cancer trends from 1972-1991 for Registered Indians living on Manitoba Reserves. *International Journal of Circumpolar Health, 57*(Suppl), 391-398.

Ross, D., Shillington, R., & Lochhead, C. (1994). *The Canadian Fact Book on Poverty 1994*: Canadian Council on Social Development.

Rothe, J. P. (2005). Towards a Better Understanding of First Nations Communities and Drinking and Driving. *International Journal of Circumpolar Health, 64*(4), 336-345.

Rozanski, A., Blumenthal, J., & Kaplan, J. (1999). Impact of psychological factors on the pathogenesis of cardiovascular disease and implications for therapy. *Circulation, 99*, 2192-2217.

Rubin, R., & Peyrot, M. (1999). Quality of life and diabetes. *Diabetes/Metabolism Research and Reviews, 15*, 205-218.

Rush, A., Polatin, P., & Gatchel, R. (2000). Depression and chronic low back pain: Establishing prorities in treatment. *Spine, 25*(20), 2566-2571.

Rutter, M., Graham, P., & Yule, W. (1970). *A neuropsychiatric study in childhood*: London: Spastics International Medical Publications.

Sacco, W., Wells, K., Friedman, A., Matthew, R., Perez, S., & Vaughan, C. (2007). Adherence, Body Mass Index, and depression in adults with type 2 diabetes: the mediational role of diabetes symptoms and self-efficacy. *Health Psychology, 26*(6), 693-700.

Saggers, S., & Gray, D. (1998). *Dealing with Alcohol: Indigenous Usage in*

Australia, New Zealand and Canada. Cambridge, UK: Cambridge University Press.

Sahmoun, A., Markland, M., & Helgerson, S. (2007). Mental health status and diabetes among whites and Native Americans: Is race an effect modifier? *Journal of Health Care for the Poor and Underserved, 18*, 599-608.

Sawchuk, C. N., Roy-Byrne, P., Goldberg, J., Manson, S. M., Noonan, C., Beals, J., et al. (2005). The relationship between post-traumatic stress disorder, depression and cardiovascular disease in an American Indian tribe. *Psychological Medicine, 35*, 1785-1794.

Shah, B. R., Hux, J. E., & Zinman, B. (2000). Increasing rates of ischemic heart disease in the native population of Ontario, Canada. *Arch Intern Med, 160*(12), 1862-1866.

Silverman, B. L., Rizzo, T. A., Cho, N. H., & Metzger, B. E. (1998). Long-term effects of the intrauterine environment. The Northwestern University Diabetes in Pregnancy Center. *Diabetes Care, 21 Suppl 2*, B142-149.

Simpson, S., Corabian, P., Jacobs, P., & Johnson, J. (2003). The cost of major comorbidity in people with diabetes mellitus. *Canadian Medical Association Journal, 168*(13), 1661-1667.

Sinclair, R. (2007). Identity lost and found: Lessons from the sixties scoop. *First Peoples Child & Family Review, 3*(1), 65-82.

Singer, M., Hopman, W., & MacKenzie, T. (1999). Physical functioning and mental health in patients with chronic medical conditions. *Quality of Life Research, 8*, 687-691.

Singh, P., Looker, H., Hanson, R., Krakoff, J., Bennett, P., & Knowler, W. (2004). Depression, diabetes, and glycemic control in Pima Indians. *Diabetes Care, 27*(2), 618-619.

Skeiky, Y. A., & Sadoff, J. C. (2006). Advances in tuberculosis vaccine strategies. *Nat Rev Microbiol, 4*(6), 469-476.

Skinner, P., & Silverman-Peach, D. (1989). Diabetes and Native Americans: Socio-cultural change, stress and copin.

Sleath, B., Chewning, B., de Vellis, B., Weinberger, M., de Vellis, R., Tudor, G., et al. (2008). Communication about depression during rheumatoid arthritis patient visits. *Arthritis & Rheumatism, 59*(2), 186-191.

Smeja, C., & Brassard, P. (2000). Tuberculosis infection in an Aboriginal (First Nations) population of Canada. *Int J Tuberc Lung Dis, 4*(10), 925-930.

Smith, G. D., Hart, C., Blane, D., Gillis, C., & Hawthorne, V. (1997). Lifetime socioeconomic position and mortality: prospective observational study. *BMJ (Clinical research ed.), 314*(7080), 547.

Smith, T., & Ruiz, J. (2002). Coronary Heart Disease In A. Christensen & M. Antoni (Eds.), *Chronic Physical Disorders: Behavioral Medicine's Perspective*. Cornwall: Blackwell Publishers.

Smye, V., & Mussell, B. (2001). *Aboriginal Mental Health: 'What Works Best'*.

Söchting, I., Corrado, R., Cohen, I. M., Ley, R., & Brasfield, C. (2007). Traumatic pasts in Canadian Aboriginal people: Further support for a complex trauma conceptualization? *BC Medical Journal, 49*(6), 320-326.

Soreff, S. M. (1996). *Handbook for the Treatment of the Seriously Mentally Ill*. Toronto, ON: Hogrefe & Huber Publishers.

Spaudling, W. D., Sullivan, M. E., & Poland, J. S. (2003). The Psychopathology of Severe Mental Illness *Treatment and Rehabilitation of Severe Mental Illness*. New York, NY: The Guilford Press.

Square, D. (1997). Fetal alcohol syndrome epidemic on Manitoba reserve, *CMAJ: Canadian Medical Association Journal* (Vol. 157, pp. 59): Canadian Medical Association.

Stanton, A., & Revenson, T. (2007). Adjustment to chronic disease: Progress and promise in research. In A. Friedman & R. Cohen Silver (Eds.), *Foundations of Health Psychology*. Oxford: Oxford Univeristy Press.

Statistics Canada (1996). Total Population by Aboriginal Group.

Statistics Canada (1999a). Low Income Cut-offs.

Statistics Canada (1999b). *National Longitudinal Survey of Children and Youth - Cycle 3*. from http://www.statcan.ca/english/Dli/Data/Ftp/nlscy/nlscy_cycle3.htm.

Statistics Canada (2001a). *Aboriginal Peoples of Canada*. from http://www12.

statcan.ca/english/census01/products/analytic/companion/abor/canada.cfm#1.

Statistics Canada (2001b). *Census 2001 Survey.* from http://www12.statcan.ca/english/census01/Products/Analytic/companion/abor/canada.cfm.

Statistics Canada (2001c). Education and learning among Aboriginal children, from http://www.statcan.ca/english/freepub/89-597-XIE/2001001/education.htm

Statistics Canada (2001d). Selected Mortality Rates First Nations on-reserve (2000) and Canada (2001).

Statistics Canada (2008a). 2006 Census Results Retrieved June, 2009

Statistics Canada (2008b). Smoking status, Inuit adults aged 15 and over by sex and age group, Canada, 2006. http://www.statcan.gc.ca/pub/89-637-x/2008002/tab/tab5-1-eng.htm

Steed, L., Cooke, D., & Newman, S. (2003). A systematic review of psychosocial outcomes following education, self-management and psychological interventions in diabetes mellitus. *Patient Education and Counselling, 51*, 5-15.

Stein, L. I. (1995). Persistent and Severe Mental Illness: Its Impact, Status, and Future Challenges. In R. Schulz & J. R. Greenley (Eds.), *Innovating in Community Mental Health: International Perspectives.* Westport, CT: Praeger Publishers.

Stephens, T., & Health Canada (1994). *Smoking among Aboriginal people in Canada, 1991.*

Stevenson, D. L., & Baker, D. P. (1987). The family-school relationship and the child's school performance. *Child Dev, 58*, 1348-1357.

Storck, M., Csordas, T. J., & Strauss, M. (2000). Depressive Illness and Navajo Healing. *Medical Anthropology Quarterly, 14*(4), 571-597.

Strachan, D. P. (2000). The role of environmental factors in asthma. *Br Med Bull, 56*(4), 865-882.

Strain, J., Smith, G., Hammer, J., McKenzie, D., Blumenfield, M., Muskin, P., et al. (1998). Adjustment disorder: A multisite study of its utilization and interventions in the consultation-liaison psychiatry setting. *General Hospital Psychiatry, 20*, 139-149.

Street Health.

Suissa, A. J. (2003). Alcoholism as a Disease in North America: A Critical Social Analysis. *Journal of Addictions Nursing, 14*, 201-208.

Sullivan, M., LaCroix, A., Russo, J., Swords, E., Sornson, M., & Katon, W. (1999). Depression in coronary heart disease: What is the appropriate diagnostic threshold? *Psychosomatics, 40*(4), 286-292.

Syme, S. L. (1989). *Control and health: a personal perspective.* : Wiley&Sons. .

Syme, S. L. (2004). Social Determinants of Health: The Community as an Empowered Partner. *Preventing Chronic Disease - Public Health Research, Practice, and Policy, 1*(1), 1-5.

Syme, S. L., & Swan, N. (1998). Mastering the control factor. Part one. *The Health Report.*, 2007

Sytkowski, P. A., D'Agostino, R. B., Belanger, A., & Kannel, W. B. (1996). Sex and time trends in cardiovascular disease incidence and mortality: the Framingham Heart Study, 1950-1989. *Am J Epidemiol, 143*(4), 338-350.

Tait, C. L. (2003). *Fetal Alcohol Syndrome Among Aboriginal People in Canada: Review and Analysis of the Intergenerational Links to Residential Schools.* Ottawa: Aboriginal Healing Foundation.

Takei, N., & Sugihara, G. (2006). Diagnostic ambiguity of subthreshold depression: Minor depression vs. adjustment disorder with depressive mood. *Acta Psychiatrica Scandinavica 114*, 114-147.

Tann, S., Yabiku, S., Okamoto, S., & Yanow, J. (2007). TRIADD: The risk for alcohol abuse, depression, and diabetes multimorbidity in the American Indian and Alaska Native population. *American Indian and Alaska Native Mental Health Research, 14*(1).

The McCreary Centre Society (1994). *Adolescent Health Survey: Chronic Illness and Disability among Youth in BC.*

Thomas, D. P., Condon, J. R., Anderson, I. P., Li, S. Q., Halpin, S., Cunningham, J., et al. (2006). Long-term trends in Indigenous deaths from chronic diseases in the Northern Territory: a foot on the brake, a foot on the accelerator. *The Medical Journal of Australia, 185*(3), 145-149.

Thommasen, H., Berkowitz, J., Thommasen, A., & Michalos, A. (2005). Understanding relationships between diabetes mellitus and health-related quality of life in a rural community *Rural Remote Health, 55*, 441.

Thommasen, H. V., Baggaley, E., Thommasen, C., & Zhang, W. (2005). Prevalence of depression and prescriptions for antidepressants, Bella Coola Valley, 2001. *Canadian Journal of Psychiatry, 50*(6), 346-352.

Thommasen, H. V., & Zhang, W. (2006). Impact of chronic disease on quality of life in the Bella Coola Valley. *Rural Remote Health, 6*(528),

Thorne, J. A. (2003). Middle ear problems in Aboriginal school children cause developmental and educational concerns. *Contemp Nurse, 16*(1-2), 145-150.

Tjepkema, M. (2002). *The Health of the Off-Reserve Aboriginal Population* (Supplements to Health Reports, volume 13, 2002 No. 82-003): Statistics Canada.

Treharne, G., Kitas, G., Lyons, A., & Booth, D. (2005). Well-being in rheumatoid arthritis: The effects of disease duration and psychosocial factors. *Journal of Health Psychology, 10*(3), 457-474.

Tsey, K., & Every, A. (2000). Evaluating aboriginal empowerment programs: the case of Family WellBeing. *Aust N Z J Public Health, 24*(5), 509-514.

U.S. National Library of Medicine and the National Institutes of Health (2005, July 2005). Medline Plus Encyclopedia Online, from http://www.nlm.nih.gov/medlineplus/encyclopedia.html

Valery, P. C., Coory, M., Stirling, J., & Green, A. C. (2006). Cancer diagnosis, treatment, and survival in Indigenous and non-Indigenous Australians: a matched cohort study. *Lancet, 367*(9525), 1842-1848.

Van Bibber, M. (1997). *It Takes A Community.*

Van Weel-Baumgarten, E. M. (2005). Is depression a chronic illness? A response from the perspective of general practice. *Chronic Illness, 1*(113-115).

Verbrugge, L., Lepkowski, J., & Konkol (1991). Levels of disability among U.S. adults with arthritis. *Journal of Gerontology, 46*(2), S71-83.

Vicary, D., & Westerman, T. (2004). 'That's just the way he is': Some implications of Aboriginal mental health beliefs. *Australian e-Journal for the Advancement of Mental Health, 3*(3).

Waldram, J. B., Herring, D. A., & Young, T. K. (2006). *Aboriginal Health in Canada: Historical, Cultural and Epidemiological Perspectives.* (2 ed.). Toronto: University of Toronto Press

Ward, E., Jemal, A., Cokkinides, V., Singh, G. K., Cardinez, C., Ghafoor, A., et al. (2004). Cancer disparities by race/ethnicity and socioeconomic status. *CA Cancer J Clin, 54*(2), 78-93.

Wardman, D., & Khan, N. (2004). Antidepressant medication use among First Nations peoples residing within British Columbia. *American Indian and Alaska Native Mental Health Research, 11*(3), 43-48.

Wardman, D., & Quantz, D. (2005). An Exploratory Study of Binge Drinking in the Aboriginal Population. *American Indian and Alaska Native Mental Health Research, 12*(1), 49-61.

Warry, W. (1998). *Unfinished Dreams: Community Healing and the Reality of Aboriginal Self-Government.* Toronto: University of Toronto Press.

Weitzman, M., Cook, S., Auinger, P., Florin, T. A., Daniels, S., Nguyen, M., et al. (2005). Tobacco smoke exposure is associated with the metabolic syndrome in adolescents. *Circulation, 112*(6), 862-869.

Wells, K., Golding, J., & Burnam, A. (1988). Psychiatric disorder in a sample of the general population with and without chronic medical conditions. *Am J Psychiatry, 145*(8), 976-981.

Wente, M. (2000). *Urban Aboriginal Homelessness in Canada*: Faculty of Social Work at the University of Toronto.

Whitaker, R. C., Pepe, M. S., Seidel, K. D., Wright, J. A., & Knopp, R. H. (1998). Gestational diabetes and the risk of offspring obesity. *Pediatrics, 101*(2), E9.

WHO (1989). *Rheumatic diseases. Report of a WHO Scientific Group.* (No. 816): WHO.

WHO (1994). Assessment of fracture risk and its application to screening for postmenopausal osteoporosis In W. S. Group (Ed.), *World Health*

Organization technical report series (Vol. 843, pp. 1-129).

WHO (1998). *Prevention of hearing impairment from chronic otitis media*. Paper presented at the WHO/CIBA Foundation Workshop. from http://www.who.int/pbd/deafness/en/chronic_otitis_media.pdf

WHO (2005a). Preventing chronic diseases: a vital investment.:

WHO (2005b). Tuberculosis Retrieved August, 2005, from http://www.who.int/tb/en/

WHO (2007). 10 Facts About Child Health Retrieved August 14, 2008, from http://www.who.int/features/factfiles/child_health2/en/index.html

WHO (2008a). Child and Adolescent Health and Development: Development Retrieved August 15, 2008, from http://news.bbc.co.uk/2/hi/asia-pacific/7562840.stm

WHO (2008b). Chronic Respiratory Diseases. *World Health Organization Programmes and Projects* Retrieved July 11, 2008, from http://www.who.int/respiratory/en/

WHO (2008c). Part Two. The urgent need for action. Chapter Two. Chronic Diseases and Poverty. *Chronic Diseases and Health Promotion* Retrieved August 15, 2008, from http://www.who.int/chp/chronic_disease_report/part2_ch2/en/index5.html

Wilton, R. (2004). Putting policy into practice? Poverty and people with serious mental illness. *Social Science & Medicine, 58*, 25-39.

Winokur, A., Maislin, G., Phillips, J., & Amsterdam, J. (1988). Insulin resistance after oral glucose tolerance testing in patients with major depression. *Am J Psychiatry, 145*(3), 325-330.

Wolfe, F. (1999). Determinants of WOMAC function, pain and stiffness scores: Evidence for the role of low back pain, symptom counts, fatigue and depression in osteoarthritis, rheumatoid arthritis and fibromyalgia *Rheumatology, 38*, 355-361.

Woolcock, A. J., & Peat, J. K. (1997). Evidence for the increase in asthma worldwide. *Ciba Found Symp, 206*, 122-134; discussion 134-129, 157-129.

Young, K., Chateau, D., & Zhang, M. (2002). Factor analysis of ethnic variation in the multiple metabolic (insulin resistance) syndrome in three Canadian populations. *Am J Hum Biol, 14*(5), 649-658.

Young, T. K., & Choi, N. W. (1985). Cancer risks among residents of Manitoba Indian reserves, 1970-79. *Can Med Assoc J, 132*(11), 1269-1272.

Young, T. K., Dean, H. J., Flett, B., & Wood-Steiman, P. (2000). Childhood obesity in a population at high risk for type 2 diabetes. *J Pediatr, 136*(3), 365-369.

Young, T. K., & Frank, J. W. (1983). Cancer Surveillance in a Remote Indian Population in Northwestern Ontario. *American Journal of Public Health, 73*(5), 515-520.

Young, T. K., Reading, J., Elias, B., & O'Neil, J. D. (2000). Type 2 diabetes mellitus in Canada's first nations: status of an epidemic in progress. *CMAJ: Canadian Medical Association Journal, 163*(5), 561-566.

Young, T. K., & Sevenhuysen, G. (1989). Obesity in northern Canadian Indians: patterns, determinants, and consequences. *Am J Clin Nutr, 49*(5), 786-793.

Young, T. K., Szathmary, E. J., Evers, S., & Wheatley, B. (1990). Geographical distribution of diabetes among the native population of Canada: a national survey. *Social Science & Medicine, 31*(2), 129-139.

Yusuf, S., Reddy, S., Ounpuu, S., & Anand, S. (2001). Global burden of cardiovascular diseases: Part II: variations in cardiovascular disease by specific ethnic groups and geographic regions and prevention strategies. *Circulation, 104*(23), 2855-2864.